Advance Praise for *Learning Sickness*

"Thank you, Jim Lang, for sharing such a heartfelt account of one man's journey through illness and back to health. Honestly, I couldn't put it down! The insights in these pages, so wonderfully written in vivid detail, bring me back through my own early trials with Crohn's disease. This is the perfect book for all people tackling chronic illness who feel they may be alone."

—Jill Sklar, author of *The First Year–Crohn's Disease and Ulcerative Colitis* and *Eating for Acid Reflux*

"In his book *Learning Sickness,* James Lang ignites an incandescent passage to understanding chronic illness. His personal path is strewn with rocks but his spirit refuses to be turned away from learning to deal with his secret pain. Sometimes truth assumes the appearance of a bitter pill, but Lang looks to a greater message when he observes 'life pulses on.' He describes a journey that is in part a search for a miracle cure, but is actually an amazing discovery of a comfort zone that waited for him all along. The reader will never hear of the 'glue' in relationships or hold the hand of a child again without a reminder of James Lang and his wisdom to look at chronic illness in its full measure and influence."

—Barbara Wolcott, Pulitzer Prize nominee and author of *David, Goliath and the Beach-Cleaning Machine*

"As a patient with Crohn's disease, I cannot help but be awed by the bravery that is so evident not only in Jim Lang's struggle to accept his illness, but also in his willingness to share his experiences. As a legal advocate for other patients with Crohn's disease, I see Jim's book as a critically important tool that will help others—doctors, insurers, government officials, and others who control the flow of resources to patients—to understand what we live with day-to-day. The worst thing about having a chronic illness is how isolating it is. *Learning Sickness* is a bridge to overcoming that isolation."

—Jennifer Jaff, attorney

"Written with clarity and honesty, James Lang's chronicle of his illness is highly informative. But Lang is intent on a higher goal as well—a chronicle of inner change and of the individual's development of a vital kind of human freedom that can discover a humble, daily but ultimately priceless meaning in life, despite—or even through—suffering."

—Reginald Gibbons, Professor and Chair, Department of English, Northwestern University, author of *Sweetbitter*

"A touching and true account of what life can be like with Crohn's disease and the impact it has on one's life . . . ."

—Annette D'Ercole, fellow inflammatory bowel disease (IBD) sufferer and mother of a child with Crohn's disease

"One of Lang's central lessons is that suffering from a chronic illness means learning to recognize yourself as a person larger than your illness. In the same way, his book is larger than a meditation on Crohn's disease; it's a manual on living a richer life."

This book explores the paradox that meditating on sickness can lead us to recognize what true health is."

—Joe Kraus, author of *The Accidental Anarchist*

"'The human body,' James Lang writes, 'does not present itself . . . as an open textbook. It is instead, like everything we find in the natural world: complex, mysterious, and capable of bursting through the categories of knowledge we have constructed to contain it.' This 'bursting through' is just what happens when Lang's own body begins to instruct him, forcing him to revise his life. *Learning Sickness* is a book about being educated in the difficult school of illness, and it points to the hard-won wisdom that may be found there."

—Mark Doty, author of *Heaven's Coast* and *Firebird*

"Chronic illness in general, and inflammatory bowel disease in particular, have found a voice in Jim Lang's *Learning Sickness*. It is a voice of wisdom, of courage, of hope, and of inspiration. You will be touched and inspired by a powerful story told by a gifted writer."

—Marvin Bush, managing partner of Winston Partners

"*Learning Sickness* is a beautifully written, frank account of one man's struggle to come to terms with the chronic illness that altered every aspect of his life. This is an inspiring and informative book that will be of value to all patients, whether they have lived with inflammatory bowel disease for many years or have just been diagnosed."

—Rodger DeRose, President and CEO, Crohn's and Colitis Foundation of America (CCFA)

"An honest and reflective first person narrative of the journey of a young professional to self-awareness and appreciation of life after being diagnosed with Crohn's disease. Written in the spirit of Anatole Broyard's *Intoxicated by My Illness*, but instead of writing about dying as an end-point, Lang writes about learning how to live each day fully. Even those who are not living with chronic illness will benefit from Lang's struggle to live each and every day. Highly recommended for medical practitioners and laypeople alike."

—Jeanette J. Norden, Ph.D., Professor and Director of Medical Education, Department of Cell and Developmental Biology, Vanderbilt University Medical School

"Lang's work is more than a brilliant description of illness; it is an articulation of health, family, and recovery. Honest, insightful, often funny, this is a book that makes you appreciate the sheer animal pleasure of being alive. Read it and experience a strong new voice."

—David Gessner, author of *Return of the Osprey*

"Eloquent and honest, this book is not merely the story of a man negotiating the specific obstacles posed by Crohn's disease and the medical establishment: It is ultimately the tale of a spiritual journey, shaped by the author's commitment to come to terms with the hard lessons taught by chronic disease."

—Michael Land, assistant professor of English, Assumption College

LEARNING SICKNESS

From *Capital Discoveries*, books that offer journeys of self-discovery, transformation, inner-awareness, and recovery. Other titles include:

Cancer Happens
by Rebecca Gifford

My Renaissance
by Rose Marie Curteman

There's a Porcupine in My Outhouse
by Michael J. Tougias

Reading Water
by Rebecca Lawton

Rivers of a Wounded Heart
by Michael Wilbur

Ancient Wisdom
by P. Zbar

Daughters of Absence
by Mindy Weisel

Wise Women Speak to the Woman Turning 30
by Jean Aziz and Peggy Stout

Swimming with Maya
by Eleanor Vincent

LEARNING SICKNESS

A Year with Crohn's Disease

James M. Lang

A CAPITAL DISCOVERIES BOOK

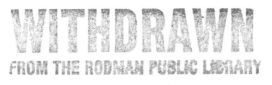

CAPITAL
BOOKS, INC.
Sterling, Virginia

Capital Books, Inc.
P.O. Box 605
Herndon, Virginia 20172-0605

ISBN 1-931868-60-3 (alk.paper)

Library of Congress Cataloging-in-Publication Data

Lang, James M.
    Learning sickness : a year with Crohn's disease / James M. Lang.—1st ed.
        p.   cm.
    Includes bibliographical references and index.
    ISBN 1-931868-60-3
    1. Lang, James M.—Health.   2. Crohn's disease—Patients—United States—Biography.   I. Title.
RC862.E52L36   2003
362.1'963445'0092—dc22   2003014801

Printed in the United States of America on acid-free paper that meets the American National Standards Institute Z39–48 Standard.

First Edition

10   9   8   7   6   5   4   3   2   1

To Anne

I suppose what I'm really to render is nothing more nor less than Life—as one man has found it.

H.G. Wells, *Tono-Bungay*

Contents

Acknowledgments

~

Of course I have many debts to acknowledge in the writing of this book.

As each chapter came fresh off the printer, it went immediately to Mike Land, who read them all carefully and thoughtfully, and provided feedback and suggestions on many levels. Once the book was complete, David Thoreen helped me refine the language with a precision and attention to words that only a poet could offer. Joe Kraus read an early version of the book, and offered several major suggestions that ultimately made the book a far more coherent piece of work that it would otherwise have been. Rachel Ramsey and Mike O'Shea read completed drafts and offered support and encouragement that I was much in need of at the time. Jeanette Norden offered me invaluable information and advice about medicine, psychology, and writing.

My siblings and in-laws all read the book in draft form as well, and to each of them I am grateful for their enthusiasm and encouragement. I have to make a special acknowledgement to Jon Roketenetz for his design of the Web site we created for the book while I was writing it, and for inspiring me with his own artistic vision and commitment. I must make an equally special acknowledgment to my brother Tony, whom you will meet in the pages that follow, and who has been—for all of my thirty-three years on this planet—a mentor and friend, as well as an older brother.

My mother and father have been and still are constant sources of support and love, and I am eternally grateful for what they provided for me on every level of existence: physical, emotional, intellectual, spiritual. Together they have modeled for me what it means to live well.

How Anne, Katie, Madeleine—and now Jillian, who is turning one year old on the day I am writing this sentence—contributed to the making of this book will be clear enough in the narrative itself, so to them I simply offer again my love and gratitude for all they have given and taught to me.

I am grateful as well to Drs. Robert Honig and John Darrah for their care of me during the year described in this book.

Finally, I want to acknowledge and thank my agent, Sandy Choron, and editor, Noemi Taylor, whose suggestions, praise, and enthusiasm for the book made me a believer in my own work.

Preface

∽

This book follows the course of a single year in my life, a year in which I struggled through a long and active phase of a chronic illness that causes inflammation, ulceration, and hemorrhaging in the lining of the digestive tract. Crohn's disease is one of many chronic illnesses characterized by the maddening habit of alternating between phases of sustained disease activity, which may last for weeks or months or even years, and phases of total remission, in which individuals may live for weeks or months or even years without any symptoms whatsoever. The maddening part is that no apparent rhyme nor reason dictates what sends the disease from one phase to the next.

For most of the year described in this book, the disease was active—more active than it had ever been in my half-dozen years of living with it, and active for the longest uninterrupted stretch I had experienced thus far. In that respect, this year represented an unusual one in the history of my illness. For some time prior to the year narrated in the book, the disease had been in remission; for six months following that year, the disease returned to a state of complete remission.

I should note that my specific Crohn's disease story, like any specific Crohn's disease story, should not be taken as a typical or general account of the disease. Every case, like every human being, is unique. Some fortunate sufferers will never experience the sort of exacerbation of symptoms that led to the hospitalization I describe in chapter six; some unfortunate sufferers will never know the joys of the remission I describe in chapters nine and ten. A majority of sufferers will have to deal with surgery at some point in their lives, a treatment option to which I have not yet had to resort.

But I am confident that most readers with Crohn's disease or its companion illness, ulcerative colitis, even if their physical symptoms and disease history vary from mine, will be able to identify with the emotional, intellectual, and spiritual reactions I had to the disease's attacks on my body. And I am hopeful that anyone who has ever confronted the limitations and defects of a physical human body, even temporary ones, will be able to identify with the lessons I learned from my disease.

Chronologically, my story in this book begins and ends in remission. In the opening pages of the first chapter I describe the final days of my life in remission, in July and early August of 2000; in the final two chapters I describe the slow return of the disease to remission, in July and August of 2001.

What I hope to convey is the evolution I underwent, as a human being, in the time spent between those two remissions. I tried to capture the essence of that evolution in the lessons I describe in each chapter. Those lessons begin, as my evolution began, with a focus on the nature of chronic illness, on disease, and upon the ways we respond to disease both as individuals and as a society. But they gradually become broader in focus, and move into more complex and universal human territories.

When I originally conceived this project, in December of 2000, I envisioned it as sociological study in which I would interview individuals with chronic illness and capture the insights and wisdom that I believed disease could offer to those of us who suffered from it. I firmly believed then—and I retain this belief still—that illness and suffering can bring a wisdom that remains unavailable to those who have not yet—and may never—have experienced them. I believe that illness and suffering can offer us insights into the most important questions we can ask ourselves about what it means to be a human being: Why do we exist? How should we behave toward one another? How do we love our spouses, and raise our children, and live our daily lives in meaningful and creative ways? I wanted this book to compile and present the collective wisdom of the chronically ill in response to these fundamental questions.

In preparation for writing that book, I sat down to tell my own story, and to think about the particular wisdom that I felt disease had brought to me. How had my responses to these questions been transformed over a year of illness and suffering? I began to write my story, and that story grew, and grew, and grew, until eventually I realized that I had all I could handle in telling my own story.

I still hope one day to write that other book, but this is the book that came out of my original intention. I will be interested to learn whether others who have undergone similar experiences with chronic illness have come to the same conclusions I have.

One final note about the book's organization.

I have tried to pin each chapter to a specific portion of the year described in the book, and those sections are arranged in chronological order—with the exception of chapter two, which flashes back to earlier periods in my life in order to provide some background on how I first learned to think about chronic illness and the human body. The dates at the beginning of each chapter identify roughly the month or season narrated in that chapter.

However, almost all of the chapters also involve movement in and out of the chronological moment identified in that date—sometimes to reflect back upon moments that had led me to the chronological moment, and sometimes to look forward to moments when incidents described in that chapter come to a close later in the chronological year, or even beyond the year described in the book. The real connecting themes of each chapter are the lessons. The time period that I identify for each chapter, then, really pinpoints the time period in which I felt that I learned that particular lesson.

I allude to each of those lessons in the chapter titles. But they are not—with the exception of the epilogue, which is a private note to my fellow Crohn's disease sufferers—offered in bulleted or numbered lists within the chapter. To offer them in that format would have made them too easily packaged, too divorced from the experiences in which they were learned, and hence too easy to ignore or file away with all of the other bits of wisdom and advice we get from our friends and our families, from the television, from our pastors, from the comic pages, and from the latest self-help craze.

I hope that the reader will see and understand these lessons as I understood them—by living through them, in each chapter, along with me.

1

LEARNING TO BE ILL

~

[*July–August 2000*]

For the record, it was my wife's idea to take in a show at the transvestite club on Bourbon Street in New Orleans. She had been trying to pull me into it all weekend, and Saturday night she broke down my resistance. Earlier that summer she had been to a transvestite show in Chicago, which had featured good-looking men in sequined gowns singing campy show tunes and 1980s hits, and she and her friends had loved it. It didn't sound half-bad for an evening of entertainment—except for the part about the show tunes—so I let her drag me into a dark and very seedy bar early that evening.

That Saturday night was our third and final evening of vacation, capping off a four-day trip to New Orleans in late July of 2000 by ourselves—no children, no other couples, no work or obligations of any sort. We were staying in a small hotel a block off Bourbon Street, and had developed a pattern since our arrival on Wednesday evening. In the mornings we slept in until noon or so, and then

1

ventured out for lunch in the Quarter. In the afternoons we would see some sights—take a river cruise, or visit the aquarium. In the evenings we had dinner out, and from dinner until at least midnight or so we would stroll up and down Bourbon Street, drinking "to go" cups of beer or rum hurricanes and wandering in and out of the bars, listening to music and watching the crowds.

More of such aimless wandering would have easily fulfilled my ambitions that Saturday night, but Anne had this better idea in mind—or an idea that seemed better to us at ten o'clock that Saturday night.

Our first clue should have been the individual outside hawking the show. He was no glamorous transvestite outfitted in a beautifully sequined gown. He had the requisite long hair and fake breasts, but he also had about fifty extra pounds for his frame, and they were shoved into a dress that belonged on a man half his size. As he winked and greeted us, I hoped that there would be no stripping.

There wasn't—there wasn't much of anything but bad singing, clumsy dancing, and the inescapable stench of male sweat mingled with perfume. The waiters were all in drag, and were very insistent about the club's two-drink minimum. In the bathroom I heard two transvestites cattily running down the outfit of a third.

The whole affair was sordid enough to be depressing, but as we stumbled out of the mercifully short show we couldn't help but laugh: that had been one *lousy* transvestite show. The bad taste in our mouths was nothing that wouldn't be cured by a few hours of strolling up and down Bourbon Street, drinking beer and listening to live music—which is how we finished the evening, and our trip to New Orleans.

It had been an absolutely idyllic vacation for us in a number of ways. First and foremost, we were on vacation alone together for the first time since our honeymoon. Even that honeymoon hadn't counted as much of a vacation. We spent seven cold and rainy January days in a condominium in Florida loaned to us by my parents' best friends, and for the entire time my wife had a terrible cold.

From our honeymoon through the birth of our first child, a period of around three years, our vacations consisted exclusively of summertime visits to our parents' homes, and trips to friends' weddings. For both sorts of trips, we were always among crowds. After our children started coming, in December of 1995, vacations on our own were no longer an option. Even when we could get family members to watch our children overnight or for a weekend, it was invariably for some event involving other people.

It took us until the summer of 2000 to con my younger sister into watching our two children for a span of four days, so we could at last have a vacation by ourselves.

As terrible as this may sound, the chance to be alone together with Anne reminded me how much fun we could have without our children, and I vowed afterward that we would continue to take vacations away from them. Despite all of the joy they can provide, children can be very difficult on vacations. Carsick, hungry, thirsty, complaining, wet-diapered, bored, tired, anxious, irritable, and inflexible—these were the adjectives that sprang to mind when I thought of car trips with our children, then ages three and five.

But the time we had alone together did not account for all of the magic of that trip. Part of it, no doubt, was New Orleans itself.

In the afternoons we usually found time to stop at the famous Café du Monde in Jackson Square, where we would drink coffee and have a beignet—a delicate French pastry absolutely smothered in powdered sugar. From our seat in the café we could watch the pedestrian traffic streaming around Jackson Square, and just across the street we could see the palm readers plying their trade at cardboard tables up and down the walkways.

One afternoon we took a paddleboat cruise down the Mississippi River, learning about the history of New Orleans and its surrounding areas from a guide as we went. We followed his monologue for most of the way, but we spent some time in the dining room as well, having a few drinks and listening to the live band they had on board. Eventually we took our drinks outside and sat near the railings on the boat's side, watching the water roll by and enjoying the gentle breeze.

Of course it was New Orleans, so the meals were a major part of the experience, and a major part of each day. We planned two touristy dinners—one at Emeril's, and one at the Commander's Palace, a restaurant that had been repeatedly ranked number one in the country by a major tour guide publication. The rest of the time we simply stopped in whatever restaurant caught our fancy in our wanderings in the Quarter. We ate plenty of Cajun food, drank plenty of beer and rum, and didn't have a bad meal all week.

One evening we settled down into a small bar to listen to a band playing Cajun music, which included a washboard as one of its instruments. I was fascinated by this instrument, the playing of which consisted of running a spoon rhythmically up and down across the slats of the metal washboard. Another evening we climbed up into the balcony of a bar overlooking the street, and stood and watched people walking by as we sipped our beers and leaned on the railing, joined by dozens of college students.

Throughout our evening strolls we would go in and out of the little shops on Bourbon Street—the voodoo shop way up at the far end, with its impossible-to-follow injunctions to take the religion of the patrons seriously; the sex shop down at the other end, where we bought a few joke gifts for friends and family; and the various junk shops along the way, where we bought feather boas and beads for our daughters to add to their dress-up collections.

And throughout all of this—in the noisy Café du Monde, over the white tablecloths of the Commander's Palace, in the gently rocking dance room of the paddleboat, and in and out of the crowds on Bourbon Street—we talked. In those four days we probably talked more than we ever had as a couple. We talked about how our lives were going thus far, whether they were turning out as we had imagined them, and what they might have in store for us in the future. Anne, an elementary-school teacher, had begun to think about a new career in health care—perhaps even returning to school for a medical degree. I was beginning a new job in a month, and had plenty of anxiety and excitement to share with her about that. We realized together how much we enjoyed traveling, and imagined other trips we might take. Our conversations were infused with a sense of hope and anticipation for the future.

"It's exciting," I remember saying to her one evening over dinner. "How wide open the future can be."

All in all, it was an incredible vacation, and by the time our plane landed back in Chicago we were already fantasizing about a return trip.

In retrospect, I suspect I may see this vacation as especially idyllic because it marked the final days of health I experienced before my yearlong descent into the heart of chronic illness. I knew I was enjoying myself while I was in New Orleans; as the year I will describe in this book wore on, I began gradually to see that time in New Orleans as the moment in which I was dancing on the cliff edge, oblivious to the tumble I was about to take. The subsequent knowledge of what I found at the bottom of the cliff slowly transformed that dance into an ever more magical and perfect time of innocence for me.

But New Orleans was not just a distinctive moment in the history of the health of my physical body; it marked, too, the final moments before I was forced to undergo some profound intellectual, emotional, and spiritual transformations. I see New Orleans now as the very last time in my life when I had been able simply to let go—to abandon thoughts of my illness, of my diet, of sobriety, of the beer and spicy food I was putting into my system, and simply enjoy myself for four days.

In New Orleans I ate and drank as I had been eating and drinking my whole adult life. When beer was available and flowing freely, I drank it until it was no longer available or until I had drunk enough to put me to sleep. If I saw foods that looked good to me, I ate them. For most of my life, I had not given any thought to the possible consequences that these behaviors could have on my body.

When I was diagnosed in 1995 with Crohn's disease, a chronic digestive disorder which causes the walls of the intestinal tract—the colon, in my case—to erupt in periodic and temporary episodes of inflammation, I was initially terrified that I would have to restrict myself to some bland, formulaic diet, eating pureed vegetables and sipping tepid water. But I quickly learned, from questioning several doctors and from research I did on my own, that—at least according to current medical knowledge—while certain foods may trigger bouts of disease activity in some people, no dietary formula or habits either cause or cure the disease. Modern medicine was unable to pinpoint precisely what caused the eruptions of inflammation in the digestive tract that characterized the disease, but it was relatively confident that food and drink played no part in it. The best current theories held that the disease was the result of an immune system disorder, and that for some reason the immune system was mistakenly directing the body to attack a non-existent foreign agent in the digestive tract.

For the first few years after my diagnosis, I saw this bit of information as a loophole that allowed me to continue my unhealthy eating and drinking behaviors uninterrupted. Of course I quickly came to realize, from both personal experience and from speaking with a dietitian, that while my diet would not actually *cause* the disease to move into its active state, it certainly could contribute to making my life especially miserable when it already *was* in its active state. In other words, diet could definitely influence the severity of my symptoms when the disease was active—symptoms that consisted primarily of diarrhea, internal bleeding, weight loss, and fatigue. When the lining of the colon is ulcerated and inflamed, the difference on the toilet the next morning between a plain bowl of rice and a bowl of rice with Cajun spices, vegetables, and sausage can be huge.

Hence I was smart enough to watch my diet when the disease was active, but when it was inactive I continued to eat and drink as I had since college—poorly and excessively.

New Orleans represents for me now the last moments of that sort of carefree eating and drinking, and that sort of inattention to the special physical needs of a chronically diseased body. More significantly, but clearly related, New Orleans also represents the last moments in which I really saw myself as distinct from my disease. Laughing in the transvestite bar, strolling along the banks of the Mississippi, eating at the lunch counters of Cajun restaurants—those were the closing moments in the first stage of my understanding of what it means to have a chronic illness, a stage that had lasted nearly five years. It was a stage in which I saw and understood disease as an external invader, as something that came from outside of me and attacked my body at occasional intervals, only to retreat and leave me alone for longer periods of remission. I was like a rebellious high school kid, and the disease was my overly restrictive parents—I behaved while they were around, but when they went out for the evening I threw wild parties and trashed the house.

IF I DIDN'T PAY ATTENTION to my diet, I did at least try to take my medications consistently. The main weapons against Crohn's disease are pills, which come in two kinds: maintenance medications, taken every day, whether the disease is active or not; and medications taken only when the disease is active, in order to help return it to a state of remission.

At the time of our trip to New Orleans I was taking two different medications. The first was Asacol, a topical anti-inflammatory, which means that it remains intact as a capsule until it reaches my small intestine, where it opens and delivers a dose of medicine to the small intestine and the colon. This was my maintenance medication, one that I will probably take every day for the rest of my life.

The second medicine was an antibiotic called Cipro, which in the wake of the World Trade Center bombings and subsequent terrorist acts became known as a treatment for anthrax poisoning. Doctors don't fully understand why Cipro (as it is commonly known) helps some patients with Crohn's disease, but it very clearly has always helped me, so my doctor prescribes it for me as a first line of attack when I am sick. About a month before we had left for New Orleans, I had experienced a slight flare of disease activity, and so I had begun taking Cipro to help calm it down. The pill had been doing its trick, but of course alcohol dilutes the effect of any antibiotic, so in that respect my indulgence in New Orleans might have helped send me down the road toward the more serious flare of disease activity that followed our vacation.

My symptoms were definitely more active when I returned home than when I had left for New Orleans, and had I been able simply to relax and recuperate for a few days I might not have ended up where I did. But as soon as we returned from New Orleans, we had to begin packing for our upcoming family move from Chicago to Massachusetts, and that activity left little time for relaxation. The transition from vacation to packing for a cross-country move probably put such stress on our systems that it would have been unlikely for me *not* eventually to have seen manifestations of it in my body. While stress, like food and drink, doesn't cause the disease, it can act as a trigger for bouts of disease activity, and it can most definitely worsen the symptoms and effects.

Stress and overindulgence in alcohol certainly nudged me toward the cliff edge I was about to fall over, but something else entirely gave me the final shove.

WE WERE MOVING because I had accepted a position as an assistant professor of English at a small New England college. I had spent the last ten years of my life, from my first years of graduate school through three years of an administrative position at my Ph.D. institution, hoping for just such a teaching position. So I had tendered my resignation to the research university where I had spent the past seven years, we had sold our tiny house in a northern Chicago suburb, and we had packed our lives into boxes.

My wife had visited our new city—Worcester, Massachusetts—several times to scout for a place to live, and we had lucked into the purchase of a spacious four-bedroom house just two miles from the college. The house was twice as large as anything we could have afforded within a hundred miles of Chicago.

Because of the children, we took three days to make the drive, stopping overnight at various points along the way. It was the last week in July of 2000, and the weather was beautiful throughout the trip. As we drove through the hilly terrain of upstate New York and western Massachusetts, we were awed by the constantly unfurling landscapes around us: vista after vista of lushly wooded mountainsides.

For the kids, the trip consisted primarily of naps in the car, sing-along tapes, and swimming in hotel pools—with the occasional fit of whining and temper tantrum thrown in, of course. For Anne and me, the trip spurred a combination of anticipation and anxiety about what our new lives would bring—new jobs, in a part of the country we knew very little about, and far removed, for the first time, from much of our families and most of our friends.

The stress factors took a definite turn upward when we finally arrived. We discovered that the previous owners of our new house had taken their washer and dryer with them, not believing them to be "fixed" appliances. We discovered that the moving company had not been able to fit all of our materials on a single truck, and that the second truck would be arriving sometime in the next three weeks. Finally, we discovered that the purchasers of our old house had been unhappy with several things they had found when they moved in—such as a nest of mice in the walls, which I can only guess we had not seen because our cat had kept them at bay—and were threatening to sue us for damages.

During the week we spent sorting all of these problems out, I made one final discovery—I had only a few Cipro pills left, and the bottle I was holding was the last authorized refill I had. To complicate matters further, I was in the midst of switching from my old university's insurance policy to the new college policy I would be on. Until the first day of school in late August, I remained on my old policy. This meant that in order to obtain a refill I would have to call my primary care physician in Chicago, tell him that I needed this medication, have him call a prescription in to a pharmacy in Massachusetts, and convince the health insurance company to pay for it. This last step was essential, since Cipro pills, at that time, cost around $7 apiece; a month's prescription ran close to $400.

In retrospect, none of those steps seem excessively burden-

some to me now; at the time, with everything else we had going
on, I couldn't bring myself to do it. I was going to stop taking the
Cipro at some point eventually, I reasoned—might as well be now.

So, with the biggest stress factor of all just weeks away—the
beginning of my first year as an assistant professor, teaching more
classes in one semester than I had taught in the last three years
combined—I took the last of my pills during the first week of
August 2000.

By the second week of August I was in the bathroom ten to
fifteen times a day, bleeding, exhausted, and depressed. I was dropping weight quickly and didn't have much of an appetite. I found
it difficult to work on my course preparations or even to help much
around the house, because of both physical fatigue and emotional
apathy.

It's not difficult to imagine how this affected my wife, who was
trying to unpack and settle a houseful of stuff, as well as take care
of our two children and find a teaching position for herself. I could
see her growing increasingly irritated with me, and increasingly
unable to handle all of the responsibility that I was dumping into
her lap. At the same time, I felt unable to do anything about it.

The arrival of my parents provided a temporary reprieve. They
had recently helped my older brother move to Connecticut, and
they drove up to Worcester to lend us a hand. My mother was able
to help assume some of the childcare duties, which relieved Anne
of some of the work. My parents also generally helped around the
house, drawing upon their thirty years of experience as homeown-
ers to help us resolve many of the little issues that arise whenever
you move into a new house.

They brought as well, of course, their concerns for my health,
which, unlike my wife's, were not leavened by frustration at my
inability to uphold my end of the household responsibilities. They

urged me to visit a local doctor, but this—like obtaining medicine—would be a complicated affair. I would have to get approval from my old health insurance provider to see a doctor for an out-of-town emergency, and then receive special authorization for any treatment I would need. Again, this does not seem like an excessively burdensome task to me in retrospect, but at the time I could not muster the energy to do it.

As the days of mid-August crawled by, bringing me closer to a first day of classes I had now begun to dread, my physical condition remained fairly stable, but my emotional state worsened considerably.

Until this particular flare-up, I had never paid much attention to the effects of disease activity on my intellect and my emotions. Looking back on the two significant flare-ups that preceded this one, it is evident to me now that I experienced the same bouts of depression, apathy, and intellectual fatigue with each one of them, but I had not yet really put two and two together. Certainly I must have understood that, when the disease was active, I had lost any desire to get out of the house, do housework, play with my children, read and write, and enjoy my life. But I attributed this simply to physical fatigue—it never occurred to me that, tired or not, I should still *want* to do these things, and that therefore some other factor was coming into play.

My inability to understand that the disease could extend its reach into my mind and my emotions no doubt stemmed from the same perspective that had been responsible for my fluctuating diet. I saw the disease as an external invader, as a biological entity that attacked my gut, and that could be fought with medicine aimed at the gut. The disease was distinct from my *self*, and especially from that part of the self that I valued most—my mind. What could my colon, after all, have to do with my emotions, my memories, my desires, my behavior—my sense of who I was?

With the semester looming and no end in sight to the disease activity I was experiencing, my emotional and intellectual state deteriorated precipitously enough to call into question this under-standing of my disease.

I felt tired all the time. I was willing to do anything to avoid spending time with my children and assuming my share of the household chores. I abandoned my writing projects. I had no desire to accompany my family to restaurants, sightseeing, or anywhere else. I wanted to stay in the house, lie on the couch, sleep, or watch television.

I could think about nothing but my disease and myself. I was able to cast my mind forward to the very next thing I needed to do or think about, but couldn't push much farther than that. I felt sorry for myself. I was convinced no one understood exactly what I was suffering, and I resented the good health of those around me. However solicitous they were about my condition, I was certain they thought I was exaggerating my health complaints.

I spent my time alternately praying for God to heal me, and resenting Him for striking me with this affliction in the first place. I rationalized not attending Catholic mass, a weekly family event, by pointing out to my mother that the bathrooms in the church were not easily accessible enough.

At some level I must have understood that this behavior was abnormal, and for a while at least I continued to mouth hopeful platitudes and express optimism about my prognosis. But this talk could not ultimately conceal my behavior—and this talk, especially, didn't help get the laundry done, or get the children to bed, or get the lawn mowed, and so on. My failings in these respects were obvious enough, and were creating a cumulative drag on my wife's patience.

One evening during the week of my parents' stay, it suddenly became apparent to me that Anne had had enough. I was tapping weakly away at the computer in the basement, working on a syllabus, and she was angrily folding laundry at a table behind me. We were exchanging irritable words about my inattention to the children, to her, to my parents, and to the household. I was feebly trying to defend myself, when all of a sudden I caught a glimpse of myself, as if on videotape, and the way I had been behaving for the past few weeks. I saw myself on the couch while she and the children headed out to dinner with my parents; I saw myself in bed while Anne straightened up the bedroom around me; I saw myself slumped in a patio chair outside while she played with the children—an astonishing rush of images of passivity.

At that moment I began crying—not so much for my irresponsible behavior, but for the realization that fully appeared to my consciousness at that moment, with all of its terrible and frightening implications. I tried to choke out an explanation to my wife's back as she embraced me, suddenly and mercifully softened by my tears.

"I think this disease is doing something to my mind," I managed to get out between sobs. "I can't understand why I'm behaving like this. This doesn't seem to be under my control."

I stayed locked in her embrace, and then we were both sobbing like children, both temporarily out of control, perhaps acknowledging for the first time that this disease had penetrated our lives in a way neither of us wanted to admit. It had become—at least in those moments when the disease asserted its control over my body—a third party in our marriage, an uninvited intruder that we somehow had to learn to accommodate.

It was a cathartic moment, and an extremely difficult one for me. That a chronic disease can have an influence on one's mind and emotions, as well as on one's physical body, may seem obvious enough, but it was a fact I had been unable to see, or had chosen to ignore, up to that point. In the basement, in Anne's embrace, I finally glimpsed this bit of illumination.

Though it had been just over a month in calendar time, I felt at that moment as if I were a hundred years from our days in New Orleans.

2

A LIFE OF ILLNESS

Learning About Disease

❧

[Diagnosis: Spring 1996; Childhood]

My illumination in the basement that August afternoon was a long time coming—much longer than it should have been. I can best explain why I blinded myself to this insight for so long by telling the stories of how I learned about disease—my own disease, and my older brother's disease, which I had lived with since my childhood.

My illness first manifested itself in the late spring of 1996, with a three-week spell of high fevers, severe diarrhea, internal bleeding, and extreme fatigue. At that time I was twenty-six years old, a new father, and a graduate student in a Ph.D. program in English literature at Northwestern University. I had completed my doctoral exams a few months earlier and had just begun my dissertation.

For three weeks during May of that year, I lay on the couch in my apartment, waiting for signs of improvement in my condition

17

and never receiving any. Before becoming ill, I had been spending two days a week watching my daughter and three days a week working on my dissertation. By the second week of my illness I was sending my daughter to daycare full-time and no longer working on my dissertation. I slept and went to the bathroom. In the morning I woke up with fevers that regularly peaked at 104 degrees, and that would never—despite a steady diet of aspirin—disappear completely.

I tried to beat the diarrhea by not eating or drinking, but it didn't help. One day I can recollect eating a single apple in the morning, and still having to make a dozen trips to the bathroom before going to bed that night. Of course the combination of the fevers, the diarrhea, and avoiding food and drink left me dehydrated, and eventually I wound up in the emergency room with such severe dehydration that they needed to pump several bags of IV fluid and electrolytes into me. My wife and daughter—our first, Katie, who was barely six months old at the time—drove me to the emergency room that night, but left when we realized that I would be spending several hours there. I took a cab home from the hospital at 4:00 AM. As I crawled into bed beside my wife, properly hydrated for the first time in weeks, I felt the first stirrings of hope I had experienced since the illness had begun. Perhaps that had been all I needed to turn myself around.

Within a few hours of waking the next morning, I was back on the toilet.

The doctors in the emergency room, like the physician I had seen after the first week, were baffled by my symptoms. I remember the emergency room doctor sitting at my bedside with a clipboard, posing question after question:

"Have you traveled out of the country lately? Eaten anything unusual? Had shellfish recently? Does your family have a history of problems like these?"

When none of his questions solicited the answers he was expecting, he simply offered me more powerful antidiarrheal medications. Those medications didn't help.

Three weeks into this illness I was finally referred to a gastroenterologist. He saw me, scheduled a colonoscopy, and at last was able to put a name to my condition.

But his diagnosis seemed impossible to me. At the most recent physical I had undergone, my doctor had run through a list of questions about my family history, my habits, and my own medical history. Setting down his clipboard, and rolling up my sleeve to check my blood pressure, he seemed almost disappointed in me.

"Boringly healthy, huh?" he said.

What could possibly explain the transition from boringly healthy to chronic disease in the space of less than a year?

Before the gastroenterologist performed the colonoscopy that eventually helped him make his diagnosis, he outlined for me the two most likely diagnoses for my condition. The first was a bacterial or viral infection of some sort, which would eventually clear up with medication or on its own; the second was Crohn's disease. The causes of Crohn's disease, he explained, were unknown. There was no cure. When the disease was active, medications could be used to help control the symptoms.

I have only one memory from my colonoscopy, which took place under a form of sedation that allowed me to remain semiconscious: at one point I asked the doctor whether he thought it was an infection or Crohn's disease. Smiling, he reassured me that it seemed to him more like the pattern of an infection.

Afterward he gave me my first prescription for Cipro, which cleared up my symptoms within a day or two, and I hoped and expected that I would soon put the entire episode behind me. Within a few days, though, the doctor called me with the results of the biopsies they had performed on tissues taken from my colon, and the news was different. It now seemed to him like Crohn's disease.

I was devastated, especially when I learned that I would now need to take medication daily, whether the disease was active or not.

My doctor softened the blow of the diagnosis by explaining to me that, at least from what he had seen during the procedure, it seemed to him like a relatively mild case of the disease, one that would probably not require hospitalization or surgery (as many patients of Crohn's disease, in the range of half to three-quarters, do at some point in their lives).

In retrospect, I see that my initial inability to come to terms with my disease, and accept its presence in my life, was seriously exacerbated by two moments from this history: the doctor's initial speculation, during the colonoscopy, that I did not have Crohn's disease; and his estimation, once he reversed that diagnosis, that my condition would remain a mild one.

For months after the diagnosis, I held onto the hope that he would again change his mind, that further studies of the biopsies, or my continued good health, would somehow persuade him that I was healthier than he had initially suspected. For at least the first year after the diagnosis, a part of me remained convinced that I could not really have the disease. I did nothing to accommodate the disease, at any rate: I made no changes in my diet; I regularly forgot or skipped my medications; I called the doctor only when I needed prescriptions refilled. I did all I could not to think about it.

Over the next several years, as frequent bouts of diarrhea and bleeding made it increasingly apparent to me that I did indeed have the disease, I held fiercely to the doctor's remark that at least I had a mild case of it. If my case were not serious, perhaps it might find its way into permanent remission? At the very least, I could hope not to suffer from the severe symptoms I had experienced during my first bout.

The second major flare of disease activity, which took place in the late winter and early spring of 1998, helped strip me of the illusion that I had a mild case.

I have two photographs of myself during the nadir of that flare. In the first picture I am in the swimming pool near my parents' condominium in Florida, throwing Katie—then three years old— into the air. She is suspended above me, in mid-toss, and we are both smiling and laughing at the pure joy of it. In the second photo I am at the beach, again with Katie, crouching in the sand and watching a young boy pet a turtle he has found. I am looking up at the camera, a serious expression on my face, squinting against the sun.

What unites these pictures for me is the shock of my naked upper frame. At the time those photos were taken, a two-month struggle with symptoms had dropped my weight from my typical 175 lbs. to around 140 lbs. In the pictures I am shirtless, wearing only my bathing suit, and the effects of the disease on my body could not be clearer.

My ribs, my collarbone, the scapula of my back are clearly visible through my skin. My face is thin and angular, my eyes are sunken, and my nose stands out against the flesh drawn tightly around my face. My head seems precariously perched on a body that hardly seems capable of supporting it. The torso in both pictures is impossibly thin and fragile, as if the slightest blow to my abdomen might crack me in half. My arms are like spaghetti—if I could step into the photograph, I am certain I could complete a circle with my finger and thumb around the upper part of my arms.

I remember standing in the kitchen one morning during that

vacation, trying to soothe my mother's anxieties about my health, to convince her that the situation was not as bad as it seemed. "Look at yourself, Jimmy!" I can remember her shouting at me, tears coming to her eyes as she jabbed at my frame with the spatula she was holding. "You can't see what you look like! You look like you've just come from a concentration camp!" When I didn't know how to respond she turned away from me and wept.

But I could not see myself at that time—could not or would not. Still desperately unwilling to acknowledge the real presence of the disease in my life, I blocked out or downplayed the significance of the weight loss, and the diarrhea, and the bleeding, and the exhaustion I was feeling. All through that flare, and the one that followed it a year or so later, I was able to remain in denial about the disease and its effects on my life.

Looking at those vacation pictures now, I realize that it has only been in the last year or so that I have truly been able to see myself as my mother must have seen me that morning, and as my family must have seen my paper-thin frame angling around the pool and the beach during that vacation—as a chronically diseased person, one whose body, mind, and life course had been fundamentally altered by illness.

The protracted and complicated process of receiving my diagnosis helped close my eyes to this reality for almost five years. But the narrative of my diagnosis does not tell the whole story of my stubborn refusal to accept myself as chronically diseased.

At the age of twenty-six, one comes upon disease with some preconceived notions about what it means, and how to confront it, and how to live with it. For me, those notions came especially from my experiences observing and interacting with the chronic disease that had been in our family for almost as long as my memory reaches back into my childhood: the juvenile diabetes of my older brother Tony, diagnosed when I was six years old.

I WAS IN SECOND GRADE at the time; Tony was in third. I don't remember what symptoms led to the diagnosis, and I don't recollect the experience of the diagnosis as especially traumatic—though undoubtedly my parents, and certainly Tony himself, would have a different perspective.

What I remember instead was how quickly Tony's disease became folded into the routines of our family life. For as long as I can remember, the laundry room in our home served as my father's "doctor's office," where he would take care of whatever small injuries had befallen his children—cuts, scrapes, and splinters, mostly. He had a basketful of first-aid materials he kept on a shelf above the washer and dryer, and he would perch us on the edge of the dryer, carefully examining and tending to our injuries.

When Tony came home with diabetes, the laundry room became the diabetic care center. An extra shelf went up over the laundry sink, one that was quickly filled with syringes, swabs, and small machines—first mechanical, and then electronic—for testing his insulin levels and his blood sugar. Sometimes I would watch Tony administering his treatments; I can remember him sitting on the dryer in the laundry room and testing his blood, giving himself shots—one day in the thigh, the next in the stomach, the next in the buttocks. I remember the pinpricks to his finger, to test the insulin levels in his blood: the click of the tiny mechanical needle, and the bright red drop of blood suddenly and magically blooming from his skin.

When I was a child, those rituals defined Tony's diabetes for me. They contributed to the sense I had—a sense that would one day color my understanding of my own disease—that his diabetes was an external invader, one that he could tame with the regular application of his needle; they contributed, more fundamentally, to my sense that the disease was not essentially part of Tony. Tony lived with our family, and shared bunk beds with me; his diabetes lived in the laundry room.

That sense of Tony as separate from his disease stemmed from other sources as well, one of which was Tony himself, and what I heard from him about his disease.

As a part of his treatment program as a child, Tony regularly visited the Cleveland Clinic for daylong programs called "Diabetic Re-Check." These days consisted of medical testing, meetings with doctors and nutritionists, and activities with other diabetic children. On at least one of these occasions, my parents sent me along with Tony for moral support—I was happy to go, since it meant a day off from school.

I don't recall much from that day except for what I realize now in retrospect was a support group meeting with a child psychiatrist or therapist, in which the diabetic children were to share their feelings with each other about having the disease. That meeting astonished me, because of the depth of feeling I heard expressed by the other children in the group. They talked about the hardships the disease had caused in their lives, and their feelings of isolation and depression. One boy actually spoke about contemplating suicide.

This came as an absolute shock to me. Tony had never expressed such feelings to me—and he and I, so near in age, were close friends—and I had never seen evidence of such emotions in him. Tony's diabetes was simply a fact of life, one more aspect of our family. In that meeting I wondered momentarily whether I had been blind to what Tony was experiencing.

Not for long. After the meeting, he joked about the seriousness of the other kids in his group, and together we laughed at the silliness of the suicidal boy. Why didn't he just suck it up and get over it?

I am certain that at least some small part of this talk, on Tony's part, was bravado, and that he undoubtedly shared some of the feelings that I heard expressed in the group that day. I cannot imagine any eight-year-old child who would not be emotionally affected by the news that he will give himself injections every day for the rest of his life. Tony simply chose not to express those feelings to me, and he protected himself from such feelings that day by mocking them when they appeared in others. He may have been in the same early stages of denial about his disease that I would experience twenty years later.

But I am also certain that Tony really did not feel these emotions, at least on a conscious level, as strongly as the other children I heard that day. I know as well that he faced his disease, as he faces it now, with far greater equanimity than any other chronically ill person I have ever known.

I have a vivid recollection of Tony and myself lounging, one steamy summer afternoon, on the makeshift grandstands that bordered one of our childhood baseball fields. Hot seats, hot sun, a childhood summer day in the middle of an endless stretch of them. Sitting with us were a few other kids from our baseball league, none of them close friends with either of us. They all knew of Tony's diabetes—he toted cans of juice and crackers with him to his baseball games, conspicuous marks of his illness, and his coaches all had to know about his disease in case of an emergency.

That day in the grandstand the other kids were eating candy purchased from the drugstore across the street, waiting for the evening baseball games to begin. For some reason that escapes my memory, the subject of Tony's diabetes came up, and then—in a sudden and inexplicable progression—their initial curiosity about what it meant for Tony to live with the disease turned into something unpleasant.

"Hey Tony," one of the boys said, waving a candy bar in his face, "want some candy?"

"Yeah," Tony replied, with a good-natured chuckle. "Very funny."

The other boys immediately joined in, holding their candy bars out to him and teasing him in the same way for several minutes.

I was furious, but helpless—all of the boys were at least a year or two older than me, and several sizes larger. I had fantasies of smashing my fist into their faces, holding their arms behind their backs and letting Tony do the same. Tony, though, seemed perfectly calm. He responded to the teasing with jokes of his own, and did not seem upset in any way. If there was a delayed reaction, it outlasted our long bicycle ride home; he never, as far as I could see, let the incident disturb him. I asked him about it recently and he had no memory of it.

At the time and even today, in retrospect, his tranquility during this confrontation was surprising to me. That tranquility remained his uniform response to the disease throughout our childhood and even to the present day: I have many memories of experiences with Tony and disease, and not a single one of them involves him showing frustration or anger or depression at his fate.

The source of his equanimity was undoubtedly my father, who refused to allow Tony to see his diabetes as a problem. Tony was simply not permitted to see, to discuss, or to think about himself as disabled or limited in any way. He played baseball, he played football, he ran track and field. He received no special treatment from my parents, at least as far as any of his siblings could tell, nor was he forbidden from any activity in which the rest of us participated.

This attitude toward physical infirmity, disease, or injury was a natural part of my father's temperament, and manifested itself in his dealings with all of his children. I remember distinctly the phrase he used, over and over again, in the face of childhood falls, cuts, and scrapes: "Tough it out." Tony toughed it out like the rest of us, despite the massive difference between our minor wounds and his major chronic disease.

What my father told my brother about his disease, and taught him to think and feel about it, helped Tony cope more effectively than any other diabetic—or any other chronically diseased person—that I have ever known. To this day, my father's impression remains in him. When I started writing this book, I had several conversations with Tony about my own disease, and about how my attitudes toward it had been at least partially shaped by my observations of his experiences. In one of those conversations, I referred to us as sharing the conditions of a "chronic disease."

"You know," he said, "I've never really thought of myself as having a chronic disease. But I guess that's true—diabetes is a chronic disease."

That he could have thought of diabetes in any other way, as anything *but* a chronic disease—one that requires daily injections and monitoring of his blood sugar, attention to his diet, and regular contacts with a physician—is a testimony to the strength of my father's influence.

In an e-mail conversation he and I conducted while I was working on this book, Tony emphasized that learning to think about his diabetes in the way he did was tremendously helpful to him. Though we had not yet discussed our shared memories of these events, he reminded me about the group support sessions at Diabetic Re-Check, and confirmed my memories of what we heard there, and his reaction to it: "You might remember some of the sessions we attended at the clinic where all these kids who could not accept their disease would sit around and talk about it," he wrote. "I remember thinking then that Dad would not stand for this, that they should just 'toughen up.' Perhaps that was insensitive on my part, but it is important in that I did not feel this to be a handicap . . . I cannot tell you how grateful I am for this, especially when I read about the difficulties that others have with their disease."

TWENTY YEARS LATER, in the face of my own chronic disease, I tried initially to "tough it out"—to apply the same principles that had worked so effectively for Tony. But I made a crucial error: My father had taught Tony to face his disease courageously, to forbid the disease from imposing unacceptable limitations on his life, and to accept it as one more of life's challenges. Instead of embracing those noble attitudes, I "toughed it out" by doing my best to ignore the disease, to pretend it didn't exist.

This was no part of Tony's or my father's strategy for handling his diabetes. Tony took his injections religiously, he tested his insulin levels when necessary, and he knew how to regulate his diet to maintain the proper blood sugar levels. Everywhere Tony went that involved physical activity—on the golf course, at his baseball games, on our bicycle rides around town—he carried with him those ubiquitous marks of his disease: a can of apple juice and a small snack. He monitored his condition, and he kept himself prepared for any contingency.

My version of toughing it out led me to behaviors in stark contrast with Tony's careful management of his disease. I ignored or downplayed the significance of early warning signs of an oncoming flare, I postponed telephone calls to the doctor and office visits when I was clearly in need of a medical intervention, and I would decrease the dosages of my medications without consulting the doctor. This was not "toughing it out," as my father defined it and as Tony lived it; this was my inability to accept the presence of the disease in my life; this was denial, plain and simple.

To live as my brother learned to live does not mean foolishly denying that disease imposes limitations on your life; growing accustomed to the necessity of daily injections, and all of the mental baggage that necessity carries with it, certainly constitutes a sort of limitation. To live as my brother learned to live with his disease, to the contrary, means not allowing those limitations to keep us from dreaming about, from striving for, and from doing what matters most to us.

To take medicines every day, to make regular contact with a physician, to submit myself to the occasional colonoscopy, to confine myself to the house or the office occasionally when the disease is at its worst—these limitations have little impact on the things that matter most to me: thinking, writing, reading, teaching, and spending time with my family.

Certainly those limitations are inconvenient, and accepting such inconveniences in my life does not come easily. I hate having to take my medicines, to spill out my pills in the morning or carry them around in my pocket when we are going out to dinner—to pull them out and choke them down, covered in pocket lint, with my dinner water. I don't particularly like visits to the doctor, and no one could possibly enjoy a colonoscopy. I don't expect any of those inconveniences to become less inconvenient with time or with my increasing acceptance of the disease; I can't imagine I will enjoy taking medicine at seventy-three any more than I do at thirty-three. But I have accustomed myself to them, and I have learned to recognize the important role they play in helping me to manage my disease.

What sent me into tears in the basement that August afternoon was the fear that the disease was encroaching upon what mattered to me most—it was preventing me from reading and writing, from caring about and attending to my family, and I had begun to fear that it would interfere with my teaching and research. And indeed, at least for a brief period, the disease had been making inroads into these areas of my life.

I reacted so forcefully because of the sharpness of the intellectual turn I had to take at that moment: from five years of denying that the disease could impose *any* limitations on my life, to the sudden awareness that it was threatening the most essential parts of myself. I was sent spinning from one extreme attitude toward disease to the other extreme.

AS I LOOK BACK AT MYSELF in that embrace in the basement, I can see very clearly what I had yet to learn: the arduous and never-ending skill of forging a life between those two extremes. Living on the extremes is the easy part: both total denial and total surrender come easily enough, for they are both strategies for keeping reality at bay. From my diagnosis through New Orleans I lived in denial; for those few weeks in August I lived in surrender.

So, having tasted both of those extremes, I was ready to begin learning the lessons that a year of illness had prepared for me. Those lessons began just a few days after my basement epiphany, where any learning about chronic illness must begin: in the doctor's office.

3

LIVING WITH UNCERTAINTY

*Learning About Doctors
and Medicine*

~

[*August—September 2000*]

My exchange with Anne in the basement helped me understand more clearly the deeper effects of the disease on my body and my identity, but it also had two more immediate and practical consequences: it opened up a better understanding and dialogue between Anne and myself, and it led to my decision to find and see a doctor immediately, despite whatever insurance hurdles I would have to leap.

Initially, the decision to see a physician gave me a great sense of relief. Once I had decided to take action, I felt confident that, whatever it might end up costing me financially, the proper medications would be able to settle the symptoms down quickly.

31

It was obvious enough to me that the solution to my problem was prednisone, a corticosteroid that doctors use for all sorts of inflammatory conditions and autoimmune diseases, including asthma, arthritis, and Crohn's disease. Prednisone, however, has serious negative side effects, both short-term cosmetic ones (like acne) and more serious long-term medical ones (like osteoporosis). It can also produce steroid dependence, leaving its users unable to get off the drug without sparking a flare-up of illness. Hence doctors generally prescribe prednisone for Crohn's disease in high doses initially to settle down a flare, and then slowly try to taper down the daily dose of the medication until the drug can be withdrawn.

I took prednisone for a year during my last major flare, most of which time was spent trying to taper off the drug, and I had been off it for a year and a half when the disease acted up in August of 2000. I knew that prednisone was what I needed, and I was confident that any gastroenterologist would agree with me. I imagined that my doctor's visit would proceed simply enough: see the doctor, explain my condition and my history, get a prednisone prescription, and wait for the flare to settle.

It's still not clear to me today whether I was being consummately naive, or whether those were reasonable expectations that were not met by the doctors I saw.

I selected a doctor by identifying one from the list of physicians available to participants in my new insurance plan at the college. That way, I reasoned, even if I had to pay for one visit, I could continue to see the same doctor I had been seeing without interruption when my new insurance kicked in. I called the office of a gastroenterologist at a nearby university hospital, and a nurse there scheduled me for an appointment very quickly when I explained the seriousness of my condition. Her reaction was a clear enough message to me that, once again, I had waited too long to take action.

When I arrived, I noticed something curious. The doctor who introduced himself to me, a man who seemed about my age, did not have the same name as the doctor with whom the nurse had booked my appointment. That first appointment proceeded in a strange sort of way. The doctor asked me a series of questions and gave me a brief physical examination. He then excused himself, and was gone for nearly half an hour.

When he returned, I noticed that he expressed his opinions in the form of the royal "we": "We feel that you need to do the following. . . . We would like you to come back tomorrow. . . ."

I realized at that point that I was dealing with a resident, and that in his absence from me he had been discussing my case with some senior doctor, and perhaps with a group of fellow residents as well. This didn't bother me much; doctors need to learn their trade, after all, and I don't mind having them learn on me—as long as they are carefully supervised by more experienced physicians. What bothered me was what he said next:

"We'd like to schedule you for a colonoscopy tomorrow. We want to take a look inside and be certain about what's happening."

"Why?" I said, trying to hide my frustration. "Isn't it obvious what's happening?"

"Most likely," he said. "But it's always possible that your symptoms could be caused by some sort of bacterial infection. We have to rule that possibility out before we can put you on the prednisone."

"Isn't there any other way for you to rule that out?"

The more I thought about it, the less I wanted to schedule a colonoscopy. School was starting in two weeks, and I was not yet fully prepared for classes. My parents were in town, my wife was still hunting for a permanent teaching position, we were readying our older daughter for kindergarten, and I didn't feel like I had time to prepare for, undergo, and recover from a colonoscopy.

The resident responded to my question simply enough: they needed the colonoscopy to rule out the possibility of an infection.

I began to babble out objections.

"I have school starting pretty soon, and my parents are in town, and I have two small children . . . this is *really* not a good time for me to do this."

"I know it's not pleasant," he said, smiling patiently, "but we really have to do this if you want us to treat you."

In other words, we're not treating you without it. No scope—no prednisone.

There was nothing I could do but agree. I thought briefly of trying to make an appointment with a different gastroenterologist, but I didn't have the energy to do that. I was in the pipeline with these doctors, and figured I might as well ride it out.

What bothered me most was the fact that my own knowledge of my body and the disease counted for nothing in this transaction. It was completely and absolutely clear to me that I was having a flare of disease activity, and that I needed prednisone to get myself back under control. In my discussion with the doctor, I had presented that self-diagnosis pretty confidently, expecting to find agreement and a prescription.

I should make clear that I do not normally diagnose my own medical conditions; if I suddenly began to have severe headaches, I would be in the doctor's office immediately, looking for a diagnosis. But living with a chronic disease is different. I live with the disease on a daily basis; nobody knows its symptoms, its patterns, its different manifestations in my body as well as I do. I will run to the doctor as quickly as anyone when something new appears, but

I had been through two flares before this one, and was experiencing exactly the same set of symptoms that I had seen before.

Subsequent events turned out to support my interpretation—I was, of course, having a flare of the disease. But the doctors did not count my interpretation of what was happening to me as medical knowledge; instead of listening to me, and perhaps calling my previous physician to confirm my history, they elected to perform a highly invasive and unpleasant medical procedure to test their own interpretations of my condition.

And perform it they did—my resident friend attending, a more senior doctor actually conducting the procedure. They almost immediately decided, once they had begun, that my colon was so inflamed that they were unable to proceed very far for fear that the scoping instrument might puncture the colon wall. So the procedure lasted less than a half hour, though that brevity did not in any way reduce the unpleasantness of the preparation and the recovery, both of which rival the procedure itself for their ability to induce physical discomfort.

Sometime during the hour or two I spent recovering on a cot in the hospital, someone handed me a prescription for prednisone. My dad and I filled it on the way home from the hospital and I began taking the medication immediately.

A week later, I had a follow-up visit scheduled to discuss the results of the colonoscopy. Once again, I was seeing the resident.

"Well, the tests for infection were all negative," he said, consulting my folder. "So you can go ahead and begin taking the prednisone."

"I've been taking prednisone since the day of the colonoscopy," I said.

"Oh," he responded. He cocked his head and gave me a suspicious look, as if he were evaluating my trustworthiness as a patient.

I could only assume that either nobody had told me not to begin the prednisone yet, or that they had told me while I was still groggy from the procedure, and it hadn't registered. But he didn't say anything else about it. The rest of the time we discussed my medication schedule and set up one more follow-up visit.

As I drove home from that appointment—on a beautiful August day, one of those late summer days that make it seem so *unreasonable* to be sick—it again occurred to me that Jim Lang had been an insignificant part of this transaction. At times it seemed almost as if the dialogue about my health were taking place between the doctor and my colon. The doctors working with me were fully aware of the seriousness of my symptoms, and of my life situation—the resident had shown a mild interest in the fact that I was a professor, and had asked me a question or two about my upcoming academic appointment. He knew that I was preparing for my first year as a professor, that we had recently moved, and that I had small children.

Nonetheless, he and his colleagues had been willing to let a week pass without offering me any treatment whatsoever—a week of a dozen bowel movements a day, debilitating fatigue, and continued weight loss. Somehow that part of the disease, the effects that it actually had on the patient's life, seemed to fall outside their purview.

Doctors are not therapists, I know. It was not my resident's job to hold my hand, help me prepare my syllabi, and talk me through my emotions. But the lack of understanding and sympathy I experienced at the hands of this team of physicians was an eye-opener for me. For them, I was a diseased colon—nothing more, nothing less.

At my final follow-up visit, to which—thanks to a babysitting mix-up—I had to bring my then-two-year-old daughter, Madeleine, I had one last disturbing exchange with the resident.

Reviewing again the results of my colonoscopy, he explained that the group of doctors who had been consulting on my case were all in agreement that my illness seemed to them more likely to be ulcerative colitis than Crohn's disease.

I knew from my own research on these related diseases that ulcerative colitis differs from Crohn's disease in that it is limited exclusively to the colon, and can be cured by a colectomy—complete removal of the colon. This doesn't work for Crohn's disease; when the colon is removed in cases of Crohn's disease, the inflammation may simply spread up the remainder of the digestive tract. Ulcerative colitis also primarily affects the inner lining of the colon, while Crohn's disease affects the entire wall of the inflamed portion of digestive tract. Apart from these subtle distinctions, though, Crohn's disease in the colon—or Crohn's colitis—and ulcerative colitis do bear a strong resemblance to one another.

The resident explained that a variety of factors suggested to them the alternate diagnosis of ulcerative colitis. I had heard this possibility before, from two previous gastroenterologists, but in the end both of those doctors had come down on the side of Crohn's disease.

I pointed this out to the resident, and noted the reasons my previous gastroenterologists had given me to support their diagnosis. The antibiotic Cipro, for example, which had always been an extremely effective drug for me, was known to work primarily for patients with Crohn's colitis. How would his diagnosis explain that?

"Well, we're not really sure," he said. "That would definitely suggest more of a likelihood of Crohn's."

"So how can you tell?" I replied. "And what difference does it make?"

"We may not ever be able to tell for certain," he said. "And in fact, around ten percent of cases of colitis can't be definitively classified, and are referred to simply as 'indeterminate colitis.' You may be one of those cases."

"So what difference does it make?"

"Not much in terms of your treatment right now," he said, "but we can ultimately cure ulcerative colitis."

"Yeah," I said, a little taken aback at that remark, "but I'd prefer to keep my colon."

"Don't worry," he said, with a small laugh. "You're not at that stage yet."

At that point he excused himself, and I waited in the tiny examination room for another forty-five minutes. Madeleine had sat patiently enough through my conversation with the resident—who had ignored her completely—but this waiting period pushed both of us to our limits. By the time a half hour had passed, I was letting her play drums with the tongue depressors, wheel madly around the room on the physician's stool, and pull yards of sanitary paper across the examination couch.

Finally a different doctor came in. He was an older man, no doubt the supervisor of the resident(s) who had been studying my case, but he made no mention of this to me, or of his role in my treatment. No one ever explained to me that I was being treated by residents, or told me who was the supervising doctor, or anything at all about the structure of care I was receiving. This new doctor had not been the physician who performed the colonoscopy; I had not seen him before in any context.

His role was apparently to put closure on my case. Because of a change in my insurance plan, it turned out that I would not continue seeing these physicians, so I had informed them that this was my last visit. This senior doctor spoke with me for several minutes about my medications, and about the future course of my treatment, and then sent me on my way.

These exchanges during my final visit with the doctors disturbed me more than any of my previous visits—though for different reasons. After five years with the disease, I had grown accustomed to doctors and their different ways of treating patients—I experienced nothing with those university physicians that I had not seen before, if perhaps in less intense forms.

What I found much more intolerable was the lack of certainty about my condition that I was forced to confront, and the realization that that uncertainty may never be resolved. It was not specifically the inability of my doctors to put a name on my condition that bothered me; I can hardly fault them for their unwillingness to make a definitive diagnosis in the face of a case that doesn't follow the rules. And I'm not sure, ultimately, if it makes a huge difference whether I have Crohn's disease or ulcerative colitis, since the treatment for both—up to the possibility of surgery—is essentially the same.

It was, instead, the way that this inability to diagnose my disease conclusively changed my understanding of the practice of medicine.

I suspect that most people come to their first conscious understanding of doctors, and medicine, at some point beyond childhood, as I did: Doctors have a definite knowledge of the human body and its potential defects and diseases, and we have only to consult the correct doctor to find the solution to our bodily malfunctionings. Certainly the body can have problems that exceed the curative powers of modern medicine, but even in those cases, such as cancer, doctors *know*: They can make clear diagnoses of our problems, they can see and understand which problems can be resolved and which cannot, and they provide the proper resolutions when they can.

One hears occasionally that many doctors have a "God complex," believing they can heal the sick and raise the dead; I suspect that this perception is more prevalent among patients, especially those who have not had much experience with doctors and disease. Our society assigns doctors especially revered places of authority and respect, and that reverential treatment depends largely upon our faith in their definitive knowledge of the human body and its ills.

The surest way to cure a patient of these perceptions is to put him in close and frequent contact with doctors trying to deal with a case of chronic illness.

My exchange with the resident on that final visit reminded me of another exchange I had—baffling to me at the time—with the physician who initially diagnosed me with Crohn's disease.

Or . . . sort of diagnosed me with Crohn's disease.

Several days after the colonoscopy he had performed on me, he telephoned me to report the results of the biopsies they had taken from my colon. Originally, just after the procedure, he had told me that it had seemed to him more like a bacterial infection than Crohn's disease. On the telephone, he explained that the tests were suggesting a different diagnosis.

"Unfortunately, Jim," he said, "what I saw in the biopsies was more consistent with Crohn's disease than with a bacterial infection."

"Okay, so . . . what exactly does that mean?"

"It means that your symptoms and tests are all consistent with what we know about Crohn's disease."

"So does that mean I *have* Crohn's disease?"

"The symptoms and tests are all consistent with Crohn's."

When I finally hung up the phone, it still wasn't clear to me whether I actually had the disease or not. I repeated the conversation to my wife, and we agreed that his strange word choice, evasive and ambiguous as it sounded to me, did seem to suggest that I had the disease. But I couldn't understand why he had not simply come out and said this: "You have Crohn's disease." Was this some strange doctor-speak, a way of avoiding medical malpractice suits in case his diagnosis turned out to be mistaken?

Looking back on that conversation from my final office visit at the university hospital, it was much clearer to me what he was doing: He was unwilling to commit definitively to a diagnosis for the simple reason that he couldn't be certain of his diagnosis. This had nothing to do with his personal competence as a physician; it had everything to do, instead, with the nature and limitations of medical knowledge in the face of this chronic disease.

Previously the relationship between the human body and its physicians had seemed to me parallel to that of an automobile and its mechanics. The parts of an automobile could malfunction in all sorts of ways, but those ways would never exceed the knowledge of the best mechanic. Whether or not he will be able to fix the problem, the mechanic will be able to identify and understand it.

What separates the automobile from the human body, of course, is that human beings design and construct automobiles; human beings reproduce other human beings, by contrast, but they do not design and construct them. The auto mechanic can always consult the manufacturer's design of an automobile to help him make his diagnosis; physicians have no such document to help them make their diagnoses.

We expect physicians to have answers. For most of my life, whenever I was ill, I viewed a trip to the doctor with relief. After seeing the doctor, I would have a clear diagnosis and probably a prescription as well. Even those people who avoid and fear seeing doctors probably do so for a similar reason—the doctor will give them a definitive explanation of their ills. The reluctant patient simply doesn't want that definitive knowledge, out of fear that the news will be bad.

Learning to live with Crohn's disease, by contrast, has meant learning to live without definitive answers, and with uncertainty. This uncertainty reaches from the very nature of my condition itself—bacterial infection or Crohn's disease? Crohn's disease or ulcerative colitis?—to the nature of the different treatments and medications that have been prescribed for me. The medicines I take at the moment are different from the medicines I took six months ago, and probably differ from the medicines I will be taking six months from now. My doctors and I are constantly tinkering with the kinds and dosages of the different medicines that are available for Crohn's disease, searching for the combination that will keep me in sustained remission. It sometimes seems to me that I am the subject of an experiment designed to determine how many different medications the human body can withstand over the course of a year.

Learning to live with Crohn's disease has meant learning to pay close attention to the physicians I see, and learning to think for myself about which tests, treatments, and medications make sense to me and which don't. It has meant conducting my own research on the disease, and keeping up to date with new developments and treatment options. It has meant learning to think for myself about which doctors can provide the different kinds of help I need.

Several years ago I was seeing a new primary care physician for the first time, and listing the medications I was taking at that time. When I mentioned one of those medications, he stopped me and asked me a few questions about it. Then he walked over to his desk and opened his *Physician's Desk Reference*, apparently consulting it for information about this particular drug. I realized at that moment that, if I needed to change my current medications or add new ones, this wasn't the doctor I wanted to consult.

But the need for me to think clearly about my disease, pursue information outside of the doctor's office, and make decisions on my own became most clear in the indirect dialogue I witnessed between my gastroenterologists and the nutritionists with whom I have spoken over the past several years.

I HAVE WORKED OR SPOKEN about my condition with five different gastroenterologists over the last six years, and I have asked each one of them the same question: "Should I be restricting my diet in any way? Are there any foods or drinks I can eliminate or add to my diet that will help my condition?"

The answer has been completely uniform: Diet has nothing to do with this disease. Eat and drink whatever you like.

This, of course, was the answer I wanted and liked to hear. Having no restrictions on my diet lessened the impact of the disease on my life.

However, in the course of conducting my own research about the disease, I have come across a number of books, articles, and people that have given me the opposite answer. Some of these sources have been diet books; some have been academic studies that suggest, for example, that consuming certain kinds of fish can help reduce inflammation in the body; and some have been nutritionists and dietitians whom I have seen, at the urging of my wife and family, over the past six years.

Anne has consistently encouraged me to see nutritionists about my eating and drinking habits, on the theory that we have to explore all possible means of treatment, and I have always been willing to do so. I view any conversation with a medical specialist as having the potential to add to my store of knowledge about Crohn's disease, about the body in general, and about the practice of medicine.

While no nutritionist or diet book has ever claimed that any one particular diet can cure my disease, or put me into permanent remission, they do consistently claim that diet can influence the course of the disease: It can help to induce remission, it can help to maintain longer remissions, and it can help to relieve symptoms when the disease is active. These claims are seductive, because they give me a sense of control: If I follow these dietary prescriptions, I can actually reduce the severity of the disease. If I listen to my gastroenterologists, by contrast, I have no such control—I remain in a purely reactionary mode, responding with medications whenever the disease becomes active.

How on earth does a layperson adjudicate these competing claims about treating the disease? I expect my gastroenterologist to have a fuller and more complete knowledge of the disease than a nutritionist; at the same time, I expect a nutritionist to have a fuller and more complete knowledge than my gastroenterologist of how diet and nutrition, at least on a general level, contribute to one's overall health. The gastroenterologists' perspective means I can eat and drink as I like; the nutritionists' perspective gives me some power to help keep my disease under control.

The dilemma of having to reconcile or choose between these competing perspectives reflects precisely what I have learned this year about doctors, about medicine, and about living with uncertainty. I have come to two important conclusions from my experiences dealing with physicians and my chronic illness: one philosophical, and one practical.

Philosophically, I have to accept that my physicians do not have the answers to all of the questions about my disease—more disturbing still, that those answers simply do not exist. The human body does not present itself to my physicians—to any of us—as an open textbook. It is, instead, like everything we find in the natural world: complex, mysterious, and capable of bursting through the categories of knowledge we have constructed to contain it. It does not obey laws or rules, it does not always respond to medications in the ways we expect it to, and it evolves and changes continuously.

Practically, this means that no one else can make my medical decisions for me. The input of friends, family, and medical specialists all can help to inform my decisions, but ultimately I have to take responsibility for them.

Consequently, all of us faced with chronic diseases need to become medical researchers, gathering as much information as possible about our bodies, our diseases, and the different treatment options currently available to us. In every interaction I have with a health care professional, I ask questions—not searching so much for answers as for perspectives. I want to understand all of the different possible ways that my nurses and physicians might be thinking about my body and my disease, so that I can identify specific treatment strategies when they are presented to me and have already thought through them. I do research on the medications prescribed for me, and read up on the latest developments in the research and treatment of my illness.

Those of us with chronic diseases need to let our knowledge inform our interactions with our doctors. This does not mean rushing into the doctor's office with the most recent newspaper articles on miracle cures. It also does not mean avoiding the doctor, and instead trying cures we read about on the Internet or hear about from friends. It means, instead, learning to make informed decisions about the care one is receiving, from choosing the right doctors to helping decide upon the best possible courses of treatment.

IN THE DIALOGUE BETWEEN my doctors and the nutritionists over the role of food and drink in affecting the disease, I reconciled their competing perspectives by acknowledging that diet certainly can help control and relieve my symptoms—if not the disease itself—and for that reason alone, I should pay some attention to it. But I also decided that I did not want to sacrifice completely the foods and drinks I loved.

So I have compromised. I place only a few food and drink restrictions on my diet, but I do make sure to eat certain healthful foods regularly, and to take vitamin supplements to counterbalance the effects of some of my medication (such as calcium pills when I am taking prednisone). This way I am ensuring that I receive the benefits of these foods and vitamins, while not forbidding myself the foods and drinks I have always enjoyed. I have also discovered recently that soluble fiber can be extremely helpful in thickening up my bowel movements and controlling diarrhea, even during moderate flares. So I eat oatmeal for breakfast every morning, and have a dose of Metamucil before lunch and dinner.

The right answers? The proper attitude toward diet and nutrition?

I wish I knew.

4

DISEASE'S ROUTINES

Learning About Daily Life

~

[October 2000]

Mornings are the worst.

Not simply because I hate getting up in the morning—which I do, and have done for most of my adult life. I am an evening person, and rarely make it to bed before midnight. I am in the right profession for this nocturnal preference. I can usually schedule my courses to begin in the late morning at the earliest, and I can do much of my schoolwork at home, on my computer in the basement, throughout the evening hours. During the school year I am often at work from 8:00 PM until midnight during the week, after a full day of classes and office hours.

However, at this point in my life, mornings have become a necessary part of my routine. My children are two and four years old, and require transportation to school and daycare; my wife teaches elementary school; and, by some bad scheduling luck, I have an

8:30 AM class two days a week this semester. So I am getting up early in the morning, at least for the fall semester.

And here's the problem: When the disease is active, mornings—and early mornings especially—are the worst time of the day for my bowels. I have to wake up at least one hour before I leave for school in the morning, to give my system a chance to excrete everything it wants to excrete before I can trust myself to the ten-minute car ride to my office at school. That may translate into as many as four or five bowel movements before I leave the house, depending on how I'm doing on any given day.

On this day in particular, a Tuesday in mid-October, I wake up around 6:30 AM. I like to be in my office at least forty-five minutes before class starts to collect my thoughts and have a few moments to gather my energy before I have to face fifteen eighteen-year-olds at 8:30, most of whom are dazed and bewildered, wondering what they're doing up so early. I wonder whether they know I hate it as much as they do.

Anne's already out of the shower by the time I pull myself out of bed at 6:45, and I stumble around her, grab my pill bottles, and spill out my morning medications: four Asacols, one Cipro, and two ten-milligram tablets of prednisone. I slug down the Asacols immediately, with a small cup of water, but the Cipro requires a full glass of water and the prednisone has to be taken with food. I carry them down with me, where I find my two daughters up unusually early, perched on the couch in front of the television. They must have heard Anne waking up and come out to find her; she must have turned on a television show for them.

I say good morning—they ignore me, transfixed by the television—and find my way to the kitchen. By the time I get there, I have to make my first trip to the bathroom. It's diarrhea, of course, but there's no blood. That's a good day. Sometimes what I want more than anything are the simplest things of all: not to have to look at my excrement in the toilet, reading it like some kind of fortune-teller for signs of an oncoming flare. I would love to be able to sit on the toilet, wipe myself, and walk away.

Back in the kitchen I pour a full glass of water, grab a banana—the only raw fruit or vegetable I allow myself to eat right now—and slump down at the kitchen table. I pop the Cipro in my mouth, gulp down as much water as I can, and begin eating the banana. When I'm finished with it, I take the prednisone, and pour myself a glass of orange juice.

I carry the juice upstairs to the bathroom with me, which Anne is just leaving. Another stop at the toilet before my shower—again diarrhea, again no blood. I feel that I might have one more bowel movement in me before I have to leave, and then might be finished for the morning. Feel or hope? Not sure.

Shower, shave, dress, and back downstairs for my morning chore—making lunch for Katie, my four-year-old kindergartner. The girls are seated expectantly at the table, still in their pajamas, and Anne is cutting up strawberries for them and making toast for their breakfast. I pour them glasses of milk and work on Katie's lunch.

Katie would make a good Crohn's patient. She eats the same bland, boring foods day in and day out: peanut butter and jelly sandwiches, macaroni and cheese, crackers, bananas. As Anne serves the girls their breakfasts, I want to reach over and grab one of the leftover strawberries and pop it into my mouth. Though I haven't eaten one in months, I can remember the taste of them—the tiny seeds, rough along your tongue and teeth, the sweet and sugary juice.

It's not worth it. I would pay for it later today, or tomorrow morning.

After the girls are finished eating I run them upstairs to help them get dressed. Two-year-old Madeleine wants to wear only dresses, no matter what the weather, and only certain ones at that, so I throw some clothes at Katie, who can dress herself, and begin the morning's battle with Madeleine. We finally compromise on a dress with a turtleneck underneath, and I help her into her clothes.

All of us back downstairs, the girls settle down for a half hour of playing before they have to leave for school. Anne and I share a few words about our schedules. Tuesdays and Thursdays are complicated childcare days, since I have to be at school from 8:00 AM until at least 4:00 PM. Anne drops both girls off every morning—Katie at school, Madeleine at her in-home daycare. On Tuesdays and Thursdays she picks up Madeleine from daycare after her school lets out, and Katie, whose kindergarten class ends an hour before Anne gets home, walks home with an older neighbor girl, and stays at her home until Anne picks her up.

On Mondays, Wednesdays, and Fridays I have no classes, just office hours from 10:00 AM to 2:00 PM. On those days I pick Katie up when she gets out of school, and together we pick up Madeleine.

I am ready to leave this morning, but stalling near the door. Do I make one more stop in the bathroom, just for safety's sake? I don't feel any urge at the moment, but that could change in a heartbeat—literally. I watch a few leaves fall from a tree in our front yard, hesitating. Up and down our tree-lined street the colors of a New England fall are in their full glory. I think for a moment how nice it would be to take a leisurely drive around the area, admiring the foliage, if only I could be assured of not having to dash off to the side of the road in search of a restroom at any moment.

I take a chance and head out the door. We live 2.3 miles from the college, a blessing for which I could not be more grateful. I barely get to the end of our street before I begin to feel some pressure in my bowels. Turn around or keep going? Can I make it the seven or eight minutes it will take me to get to school?

I press onward.

Almost a mistake. Some traffic at the intersection of the grade school I have to pass slows me up, and when I finally pull into the parking lot the pot is nearly boiling over. I dash into my office, throw my stuff into a chair, and make it to the bathroom just in time. The stalls around me are empty at this time of the morning, and it's a relief to be at school, so I relax and take my time. Colleges are wonderful places for people with Crohn's disease to work—public restrooms everywhere you turn. I'm never more than a few hundred yards from a toilet.

Anne firmly believes that my close calls in the car, which happen frequently, are a psychological phenomenon—that every time I get into a car I suddenly have to go to the bathroom, because I am paranoid about finding myself stuck away from a public restroom. The fact that I almost always—though there have been a few notable exceptions—make it to a restroom on time would support that theory. I don't doubt that Anne is correct, but even if the source of the pressure on my bowels is psychological it doesn't make it any less real, or any less insistent.

Back in my office I pull out the small scrap of paper I have been carrying around with me for the past two weeks and write today's date on it, along with the times of each bowel movement I have had that day. I mark a small notation, "NB"—no blood—next to each of them. The scrap of paper is covered with tiny, cryptic writing: the dates for the past two weeks, under which stretch long columns of times: 7:00 AM, 7:20 AM, 8:00 AM. The columns, at this point, are mostly five to seven entries long. I have had columns that stretch into the high teens.

One of the best weapons against disease, I know, is information. The more information I have about what constitutes normal for my body, the more quickly I will be able to identify deviations from that normalcy, and know when to seek treatment. So I should keep these notes all of the time—instead of, as I do, in clumps of two- or three-week periods, saved on random scraps of paper I shove into my wallet or drop into my desk drawer at work.

Although I know I should keep this notebook constantly, I find I can only tolerate it for so long. At some point, seeing the columns slowly fill the piece of paper begins to depress me, so I toss the note into a file folder I keep on the disease and prefer to live in ignorance for a while.

In the office I settle in at my desk, check my e-mail, and prepare some handouts for class. At 8:15 AM I am ready for one last trip to the restroom when a colleague stops into my office for a chat. She has nothing in particular to say, just idle chatter. Given the solitary nature of the academic life, these interoffice visits are often the only opportunity we have for conversation with other adults during the workday.

But as the chatter stretches on, the pressure on my bowels begins to increase. I hold, clench, breathe slowly, and begin fooling around with papers on my desk, hoping she'll get the message that I need to excuse myself.

If my disease were public knowledge, I could easily interrupt and tell her what was going on. But thus far—two months into my first semester—I have decided to keep my disease a secret. Part of that stems from not wanting others to see or treat me differently; the other part stems from the socially embarrassing nature of the disease's symptoms. Somehow I find it difficult to tolerate the thought of excusing myself from a conversation or a meeting, and knowing that everyone in the room is wondering if I am running off to have a watery bowel movement.

Eventually I tell her that I have to leave for class—this she can certainly understand—and I gather my things and take them with me for one last trip to the restroom.

After four or five bowel movements since I have been awake this morning, I can tell I am getting dehydrated. My mouth is dry, and I feel slightly shaky. I get a bottle of water from the vending machine near my classroom.

In class—freshman composition—the students are workshopping first drafts of an essay, which means they sit in circles of three or four and exchange their papers, reading one another's work and responding to a series of questions that I have designed for them.

In other words, easy day for me. However, I usually have to spend ten or fifteen minutes beforehand going over course business—upcoming due dates, changes to the syllabus, announcements for one or another event sponsored by the department—and preparing the students for the exercise.

About ten minutes into this preparatory patter—no surprise—I begin to feel some pressure on my bowels once again. I speed up my delivery. If I can make it through a few more minutes, I will be able to run to the restroom across the hall while they work on one another's papers. Pressure builds slowly, and I think about making a dash for it before I have even finished, but then it lessens for a few moments. I finish up my comments, see that they have begun reading one another's papers in earnest, and get to the restroom with time to spare.

While I'm there I feel gratitude again that I teach at the college level, in classrooms which one can leave unattended for a few moments without fearing that the students will burst into riots or destroy the room.

Sometimes I run through different professions in my head, wondering which ones would be the most difficult for a person with Crohn's disease—for a person, more plainly, who regularly has to make sudden and urgent trips to the restroom.

Best jobs for Crohn's disease: any job in a big office with large, anonymous restrooms—though it should be a lower-level position that does not involve spending an excessive amount of time at high-pressure meetings; any sort of freelance creative work; any job that one can do at home; health professional (hospitals and doctor's offices are chock-full of bathrooms); hotel employee (ditto); and, of course, restroom attendant.

Worst jobs for Crohn's disease: sales (lots of traveling and meetings with people); sole proprietor of a store; airline pilot; professional athlete; Wall Street trader ("I had to run to the restroom, and I lost my firm $100,000"); and, perhaps worst of all, surgeon ("Nurse, put your finger right here and press down until I get back").

In class everything winds down smoothly, and I finish up the rest of the morning without incident.

Back in my office, I settle into the easy chair I bought at the Salvation Army and allow myself a few moments of depression. It has been a bad morning. Close calls on the way to school, in my office, and in the classroom.

Close calls always intensify my feelings of stress and depression about the disease, because not all close calls are happily resolved. The offices in my department are in former dormitory rooms, and each office has a student wardrobe in it. In that wardrobe I keep an extra pair of shoes and a complete change of clothes, in case I don't make it to the toilet on time.

This has not happened to me more than a handful of times, but each instance of it sends me into a spiral of depression. It is almost impossible to convey to the uninitiated the full sense of degradation, shame, and humiliation one feels after an accident like that.

The most recent accident I had occurred with only one witness—my youngest daughter, Madeleine, who never even knew that it had happened.

IT HAPPENED ONE FRIDAY early in the fall semester, when I had no classes and had elected to keep Madeleine home with me instead of sending her to her daycare provider. I had planned a trip to a nearby mall to purchase birthday presents for my wife.

I waited until nearly 10:00 AM to leave, wanting to ensure that my bowels were completely emptied for the morning. When we finally took off I was confident that everything was fine, and the two of us set off in high spirits, singing along to one of her tapes of children's songs.

Not five minutes into the ride—just, of course, as I was pulling onto the highway—I felt a sudden wave of pressure. I thought I could hold on until we made it to the mall, which was a mere fifteen minutes away. I didn't have much choice, at any rate—we were still new to the area, and I didn't know the highway exits well enough to locate a public restroom quickly if we did exit.

Five minutes into the ride, the situation had begun to reach crisis point. No exit signs were in sight, and along the side of the road—the absolute last resort for a desperate Crohn's patient— there was no shoulder and no tree cover. On either side of the traffic lanes were thin shoulders, concrete barriers, and sheer drops down into a valley below. I couldn't just pull over, and even if I could I would have had to take care of my business in full view of all passersby.

I did my best to hold on, but it is literally impossible to hold material in your bowel when it is inflamed and bloodied; the body eventually will force it out, as it did at that moment. Some newspapers were lying on the passenger seat, and I reached for these and put them under myself to preserve the car seat as best I could. Usually releasing only a small amount will relieve the pressure, so I wasn't exactly swimming in the stuff, but it was enough to make me uncomfortable. I pulled off at the first exit, and got back on the highway heading for home.

Twenty very long minutes later, I pulled into my driveway. Madeleine had fallen asleep. I glanced at the neighbor's house and saw no signs of life, so I ran quickly from the car, through the garage, and into the laundry room. I stripped, wiped myself down, and found a dirty pair of sweatpants on the floor. I put them on, retrieved Madeleine from the car and deposited her—still sleeping—on the couch, and took a shower. In the shower I couldn't help but cry a little bit, feeling sorry for myself. It was part shame—Why?—part relief—What if one of the neighbors had seen me? What if it had happened in the middle of a store at the mall?—and part frustration and rage at the hand I'd been dealt.

To sit in your own shit is to come face-to-face with the ugliest part of yourself and your body, and to be given a visceral reminder of the disease's power to control your life. I can ignore my diet, I can refuse my medications, I can even choose to end my life if I want—but when that stuff has to come out, it comes out, whether I want it to or not. No choice; no free will; no control.

This is a jarring lesson to receive on a sunny Friday morning in September on the way to the mall—jarring at any time, I suppose.

The one blessing buried in the experience was that Madeleine never knew that anything unusual had happened. She never even asked me why we didn't make it to the mall.

I SHOULD TAKE A LESSON from Madeleine's obliviousness, but instead—back in my office easy chair on this sunny October morning—I replay the incident over and over again in my mind. The thought of that day still incites feelings of shame and humiliation, and my mind hovers around the memory the way the tongue endlessly probes a canker sore. It is the sort of memory that one tries to shake off with a jerk of the head, but that lingers on, floating in some place in my mind that I can't seem to close off.

On the positive side, I feel a certain amount of gratitude that I made it through this particular morning without such an incident.

That sense of gratitude may be one significant thing that separates the chronically diseased from the rest of the population—we can be grateful for the smallest of life's gifts. You can't truly appreciate a solid bowel movement until you've gone six months without one. You can't truly appreciate a public restroom until you've shat yourself for want of one.

I fill the remaining hour or so until my next class doing one of the few things that makes me feel better about the disease— reading the stories of others who share my problems on one of the many Web sites devoted to Crohn's disease and ulcerative colitis.

I find a good one this morning:

> Traveling to England as a professor for an adult oriented college trip, I suffered intense flare-ups from my newly diagnosed Crohn's Disease. My good friend, the director of this Lutheran University, and I were chaperoning students to Bath, England. During the morning of sightseeing many cathedrals, I felt the intense urge to find a restroom. Vicki, knowing my condition, started looking for a WC (water closets as they are called in Europe). I am now running through the streets of Bath, deserting the students in the cathedral—un-chaperoned. Vicki and I find a pub—I proceed to make the WC my home for the next 1/2 hour. When I finally arrive out of the WC, I find my friend Vicki, having a 1/2 pint at the pub's bar. You see the owner of the pub demanded that only patrons could use the restroom,

and that since I was a rude American running into the bathroom, she had to purchase something from the pub. What makes this story interesting is that it was 9:00 in the morning and the students were all standing in the doorway looking for the two chaperones and finding us having a beer.

This post comes from one of my favorites: the IBD Humor Page.* Compiled by a sufferer of Crohn's disease, the site contains the stories of dozens of people who have found themselves in situations as—or more—embarrassing than any I have ever experienced. Knowing that others share the same tribulations brings a comfort of sorts. The professor's story brings me particular reassurance because I have recently agreed to co-chaperone a group of students to Ireland for spring break next year.

But in general, the contributors to these pages have learned a lesson that took a couple of years to sink in for me: It's hard to take oneself too seriously when you've sat in your own shit as an adult—and on more than one occasion.

Revitalized and comforted by the stories of others—and another dose of Asacol working its way through my system—I have a fantastic class in contemporary British fiction, in which we are reading and discussing Grahame Greene's novel *The End of the Affair*. Near the end of the novel the main female character takes ill in one of those unspecified, novelistic ways. She has a cough, and becomes weak and feverish, and then dies in her bed. How glibly a novelist can gloss over the painful details of illness! It makes me wonder whether Greene ever came into close contact with real illness—if he had, I'm not sure he would have been so willing to use the character's illness, killing her off with a cough and a fever, to provoke some self-reflection on the part of his male narrator.

*This site was no longer active at the time this book went to press.

I found this tendency on the part of writers about illness especially frustrating during the few years between the time I was diagnosed and the time I discovered Web pages like the IBD Humor Page. I would read about cases of Crohn's disease patients in published books who would describe their troubles with easy euphemisms: "I was having a lot of GI trouble at that time. . . . My stomach was really acting up. . . . I was having a lot of discomfort in my abdomen. . . ."; or, the blandest of all: "I was sick."

What do you mean by that? I wanted to shout to the books I was reading. Have you soiled your pants like I did? Have you spent twenty awful minutes on the toilet, and then stood up and looked into the bowl and seen your own bright red blood? Have you lain in bed late at night, knowing that inside you somewhere, in a place you can't reach and can't control, blood is leaking from your intestines? Have you lain in bed late at night and wondered whether the disease is slowly burning holes into the wall of your intestines as it sometimes does? Have you lain on the couch for hours and even days, trotting back and forth to the restroom every ten minutes until you were too weak to get up anymore? Have you, in other words, been through what I'm going through? For a few years I wondered whether anyone else in the world could understand my experiences.

The stories I discovered on the Web taught me that, all things considered, I was much better off than many Crohn's patients, who often must deal simultaneously with a host of complications from their symptoms (such as fistulae, which occur when the disease burns a hole through the wall of the intestine and into a nearby organ), with surgeries, and with related autoimmune disorders (skin rashes, joint and muscle pains, other digestive problems). They also helped me see that others did in fact have the same experiences as I did. As I will discuss in more detail in chapter eight, those discoveries slowly helped me see my way to sharing my own story with others.

AFTER CLASS, reveling in the afterglow of seventy-five minutes of stimulating intellectual discussion, I realize again how profoundly this disease affects my thinking about just about everything. Four years ago I would have read *The End of the Affair* and not given one iota of thought to Greene's descriptions of illness.

I have lunch with a few fellow professors, and eat my regular meal in the cafeteria—a chicken wrap with mushrooms. I usually see any vegetables I consume in the toilet the following morning, but my system seems to tolerate mushrooms fairly well.

At 2:30 in the afternoon I do a reprise of the morning composition class, though without the close calls. This group of students is fun, and I enjoy myself.

I pick up a few things from my office, check my e-mail one last time, and head for home. My system has settled down by this point, and I have the luxury of a few hours without worrying about my bowels. Usually—at least during this current flare—I can feel comfortable that I will be able to keep things under control from around noon or so until seven or eight o'clock in the evening.

So when Katie and Madeleine clamor for a trip to the park a few blocks away, I agree to take them there for an hour or so before dinner. On the way down the hill over which our street passes we run into a neighbor playing outside with her children, and she decides to join us. The group of us walks together to the park.

Once there, I sit down with my neighbor for a few minutes on the bench while the girls attack the playground equipment with relish. My neighbor and I exchange pleasantries, talk about the children, about other happenings in the city. But we run out of pleasantries quickly enough—and I've never been much of a pleasantry person at any rate.

So in a few minutes I'm off the bench and I'm doing what I do best at the playground—playing. I start up a game of freeze tag, which the older kids on our street have just discovered, and volunteer to be "it" for the first time. A few other kids we don't know, supervised by bemused parents on the benches, join in.

Within a few minutes the air is filled with the squeals of mock-scared little girls, the thumping of feet on the play structure's suspended wooden bridge, and my mock-threatening growls. I chase the kids all around, just missing them at every turn, and I wonder if they realize I am letting them go, and it's all part of the fun, or do they really believe they are quicker than me?

I get lost in the play, in the pure enjoyment of body movement and the careful negotiation of the rules of the game, in the desire to help these small human beings experience these moments of pleasure as intensely as I do. Madeleine doesn't understand the game, she runs from me and squeals if I tag her, following the nearest older children to whatever point of safety they have managed to obtain.

Eventually I wear myself out and gather the girls away from their friends and the playground, and we make our way slowly back to the house, to Anne, to dinner, to the remains of the day.

AFTER DINNER I get a phone call from one of my neighbors, a child psychiatrist who lives three houses down and has a daughter the same age as Madeleine. He has tickets to a Celtics game, he tells me, which include a complimentary buffet dinner and free drinks beforehand inside the Fleet Center. All we have to do is sit through the lecture of some professor talking about a new drug for psychiatric illnesses. I learn later that this is a common practice. Drug companies sponsor events or dinners for practicing doctors to which they invite professors or researchers to come and speak about their products.

I am not an especially big fan of the NBA, but in general I enjoy live sporting events, and the free buffet dinner and beer make this invitation especially enticing.

But I hesitate nonetheless. The game is two weeks away, on a weeknight, and the Fleet Center—the home of the Boston Celtics—is forty-five miles from our house in Worcester.

"We're going to drive in to the train station," my neighbor tells me, "and take the train to the Fleet."

I work out the details. A forty-five-minute drive in rush-hour traffic, followed by another thirty-minute ride on the train. Repeat in reverse order for the trip home.

I wouldn't mind the drive so much if I were by myself, but with other people in the car it becomes complicated. Do I want to chance having to suddenly jump out of the car, in rush-hour traffic, and bolt to the side of the highway to relieve myself? The train presents an equally disturbing prospect—what if the urge overcomes me on a long stretch between stops? What if I have to jump off the train at an unfamiliar stop?

These sorts of calculations are so routine to me now that my mind runs through them automatically whenever I contemplate traveling anywhere.

In this case, I decide that my potential enjoyment of this experience outweighs the possible risks, and I agree to go. As often as not, though, I will decline and elect to stay home, unwilling to take the chance of finding myself stuck somewhere, in a public place with strangers or even friends, without a restroom.

WE FINALLY BUNDLE the kids off to bed at around 8:00 PM, and Anne immediately changes into her pajamas and settles onto the couch for some television. She'll be asleep within an hour. Chasing around twenty-some seven-year-olds, and then coming home to chase our two- and four-year-old doesn't leave her much energy for weekday evenings.

Not that it matters much to me during the school year. I bolt immediately for the basement computer, and begin a marathon session of responding to the student drafts I received from my two composition classes earlier this morning. It takes me around fifteen minutes per draft, which means—with the occasional break—I can get to perhaps twelve of them this evening.

As 11:00 PM approaches, I can feel my concentration begin to sag, and I find myself surfing the Internet, checking a few Web sites on college football and reading up on the coming weekend's games. When I officially give up and log off a few minutes after eleven o'clock, I've only made it through ten papers. Twenty-one more will be waiting for me tomorrow morning.

I take my evening medications, pour myself a beer, and settle down to watch a rerun of *The Simpsons*. I drink two more beers before I make it to bed around midnight.

Beer, as my mother and wife have been reminding me for years, is no part of the ideal Crohn's disease diet, and I wouldn't recommend it to any fellow sufferer. In chapter nine I will describe in more detail the lesson I learned about the role that alcohol had been playing in my life, and the steps I took to modify that role.

But I haven't learned that lesson yet. So the last hour of my evening, in which I usually watch television and have a couple of beers—and have been doing so for the past ten years—represents the one part of my day when I absolutely don't worry about my health. Sitting on the couch, drinking beer, I feel like I'm in college again, before all of this started—healthy, normal, enjoying my physical self. Back to the days when I had never heard of Crohn's disease, and any diarrhea I experienced was just from the cafeteria food.

In bed a little after midnight, I look at the clock. Do I need to set the alarm? No teaching tomorrow. Anne will wake me up when she needs help with the girls.

REHEARSING THE ROUTINES of daily life reminds me how deeply the disease penetrates my existence—how much of my days are devoted to wondering where the next restroom might be, or worrying about how I'll be feeling in two weeks at the Celtics game, or in one year when I'm in Ireland, or thinking about any of the myriad effects of the disease in my life. If someone who could gain access to my brain offered me a minute-by-minute breakdown, I would ask them not to tell me what they had discovered. Learning how much of my life and my intellectual energies get nibbled away by the appetite of the disease would only depress me.

In the routines of daily life—interrupted, transformed, pocked, and staggered with medication schedules and trips to the restroom—the disease makes its presence felt most deeply. As I rehearse those routines, and lay them out on paper, I see how fully I am forced to build my life around the disease—how it determines and controls so many parts of my existence.

But I have learned that building my life around the disease beats the alternative: planning and living my life as if the disease didn't exist, and then suffering the consequences when it reacts and disrupts my life in ways I haven't anticipated. The disease may close off certain possibilities to me, but I would rather shut those doors myself at the outset than have them slammed on me when I have already stuck my nose in. And, in sometimes unexpected ways, as I will describe in later chapters, the disease may open other possibilities.

A life built around disease is still a life. Like almost any other life, the possible paths along which it might unfold are not endless, and are bounded by limitations and constraints. A clear-eyed, realistic understanding of the borders and obstacles of my path—an understanding that came for me only when I began to describe them on paper—may be the best tool I have to negotiate it successfully.

5

SMALL MIRACLES

Learning About God

[*November–December 2000*]

The Christ I read about in the Bible—a Bible I know from thirty years of Catholic masses, from Catholic school education from first grade through my M.A. degree, and from several personal readings of the New Testament during Lenten seasons—responds to human suffering and illness in a uniform manner: He heals the sick. Lepers, blind men, deaf men, epileptics, a woman with a skin affliction, men and women possessed by demons, Lazarus, the daughter of the Roman centurion, a paralytic, a man with a withered hand. When Christ meets suffering, he responds with healing.

He tells us, too, that we have only to believe in Him, and ask, and our prayers shall be answered: "Ask, and it will be given to you; search, and you will find; knock, and the door will be opened to you. For everyone who asks receives; everyone who searches finds; everyone who knocks will have the door opened" (Matthew 7:7).

For five years now I have been knocking on that door; I'm still waiting for it to open.

IT IS A COLD DECEMBER DAY, at the edge of the semester's close, and I lock my office door and trek out into the lightly blowing snow, across the campus toward the college chapel. The walk isn't long, perhaps a few hundred yards. Still, I take it slowly, testing whether the walk will loosen up my system and send me sprinting back to the bathrooms in my office building. The chapel has no bathroom in it; I asked someone, of course, the first time I attended a mass there. I always ask.

The chapel is warm and welcoming. Soft lighting lies upon the long, arched wooden beams stretching up to form the roof of the building. Behind me the rays from a clouded winter sun filter through the stained-glass rear window of the chapel.

It is quiet enough in the chapel that the smallest rustlings, the most discreet coughs, are amplified throughout the large and near-empty structure. An elderly gentleman—I've seen him at every noon mass I've attended—greeted me when I came into the back of the chapel. Scattered throughout the pews are perhaps eight other mass-goers: most of them elderly, from the neighborhood around the college. I see one middle-aged woman who might be faculty or staff. No students.

Next to the altar the priest sits quietly, dressed in the purple robes of Advent, his hands folded in his lap. He seems absorbed in thought, or perhaps prayer.

The bell outside the chapel rings twelve times, and the priest stands and raises his arms, signaling for the dozen of us in the pews to follow his lead.

Mass has begun.

SINCE THANKSGIVING, when we had spent five days in St. Louis visiting Anne's parents, my illness had been steadily worsening. From four or five bowel movements a day through most of the fall, I was edging up to seven or eight, with spots of blood here and there, and an increasing number of close calls. I was staying at home or in my office as much as possible, venturing away from familiar restrooms only if it was absolutely necessary. Worst of all, I could feel myself just beginning the slow slide into depression that had overtaken me in August.

I had been trying to taper off prednisone throughout the fall semester and it hadn't been working. I could reduce from forty to thirty to twenty milligrams without much trouble, but every time I dipped below twenty milligrams per day the disease became active almost immediately. I would ratchet the dosage back up until I settled down and then try again. In late November I went through the same cycle, but this time, when I ratcheted myself back up to the higher dosage, I didn't settle down.

I was a little smarter in late November than I had been in August, and in early December I made an appointment with the gastroenterologist I had begun seeing after I switched from the university doctors. I was hopeful that an earlier intervention might produce better results.

The first time I had met with this new gastroenterologist, in October, we had discussed the possibility of my starting Imuran, an immunosuppressive medication that was becoming increasingly common for Crohn's disease treatment. Imuran had been developed initially for kidney transplant patients. It suppressed their immune systems after surgery, preventing their bodies from attacking the foreign organ. In much smaller dosages, the drug had been tested on patients with Crohn's disease, and had shown remarkable results. I had heard reports of patients with disease patterns similar to mine, or worse, enjoying remissions for as long as four or five years.

The university doctors had strongly recommended that I begin taking this drug, as had my gastroenterologist in Chicago during my last visit with him in the spring. I had demurred on those occasions, for the not-very-good reason that I didn't want to add another drug to the small pile of daily pills I was already taking. I did not think through the prospect enough to realize that, should the Imuran work for me, it would allow me to reduce or eliminate some of those other medications.

I had learned along the way that Imuran also has helped taper patients off steroids. So by the time I saw my new GI in October, I was ready, and I told him so.

"I'd like to hold off on that for a little bit," he said to me initially, to my surprise.

"Why?"

"Since I have not seen you before, I want to see how you respond to the more conventional medicines first, and get a sense of your disease pattern. I know that Imuran is becoming more popular as a first-line medication for Crohn's patients, but I view it with caution. This is a serious drug."

"What do you mean?"

"I mean that we are still learning about its potential side effects. There have been some cases of lymphoma associated with the disease. It can render you more susceptible to infections and contagious diseases. And are you planning on having more children?"

We were.

"There may be risks of birth defects."

I was taken aback by this, and must have shown it.

"I don't want to scare you," he continued. "The number of

cases of lymphoma is rare enough that they have been written up
in medical journals. And we don't really know for certain about the
effects of the drug on the reproductive system. But I want us to
approach it with caution. It is a serious drug, and we should use it
in serious circumstances. I am not convinced you're there yet."

So we had agreed to wait. But as the semester drew to a close,
and my condition began to worsen gradually, I had been rethinking
that decision. When I made the appointment with him in December, I was certain that I should begin the new drug.

But on the day I went into his office I was having a good morning, feeling stronger than I had been recently and my bowels
slightly more under control. Even though I know perfectly well that
one can't make any judgments about the disease based on a single
day, I can't help but be affected by especially good and bad days.

So in the doctor's office in early December I hemmed and
hawed, and he hemmed and hawed as well. Finally we agreed that,
with four weeks of semester break coming up, I would have time
to relax, to sleep, and to heal. We would see if I improved over
break; if I didn't, we would begin the new medication in January.

That good day—of course—had been followed by a bad one,
and I had not been improving at all in the days since my appointment.

IN THE CHAPEL I was settling into the routines and rhythms of
the mass: the welcoming, the opening prayers, and then the readings of the gospels. For some silly reason, I had an expectation that
God would speak to me through the Gospel reading that day—that
it would be a story of suffering and healing, meant to comfort me.

It wasn't. I can't even recall what the reading was about anymore, but I remember feeling disappointed that it didn't apply to
me. I listened to it, and to the brief sermon of the priest that

followed. In that sermon, I waited for a special message from God, through the mouth of the priest. Again, nothing.

I have never been much enamored of the mechanics of the Roman Catholic liturgy. I know Catholics who find the mass an inspiring and aesthetically pleasing spectacle; they kneel devoutly and ecstatically before the risen host at the celebration of the Eucharist, their hearts lifted by the thought that Christ's body will enter their own.

I am not one of those people. I have always struggled through mass. My mind wanders, my knees and butt get sore, and I spend much of my time watching the activities of my children, or of other small children around me. I generally listen to the Gospels, and the homily, and find material for reflection in those parts of the mass, but I spend very little time in mass praying in the way that I suspect those around me are doing.

I go, though. I've been going since I was born. I skip mass a little more frequently these days than I did when my parents herded us all there every Sunday of my childhood, but even now, more often that not, Sunday mornings will find me in church.

I am reminded of my long and familiar association with the mass as the priest recites parts of the mass that I have—without thought, through sheer volume of repetitions—committed to memory:

"Lord Jesus Christ, you said to your apostles, my peace I give to you, I give you my peace. . . . Look not on our sins but on the faith of your church as we wait in joyful hope for the coming of our savior, Jesus Christ. . . . Let us all share with one another a sign of Christ's peace. . . ."

At this signal to greet my neighbors in the pews and offer them the sign of peace, I look around rather futilely at the empty rows separating me from the nearest human being in the chapel. I receive a few nods and smiles from afar, and flash a two-fingered peace sign to a woman across the aisle from me.

This brief interlude of social interaction within the mass concluded, the priest begins the rituals of blessing and preparing for the celebration of the Eucharist.

WHEN I REFLECT upon the literally thousands of masses I attended while I lived in my parents' home, what stands out for me are feelings of warmth and comfort, both of the familial and spiritual kind.

No doubt I have telescoped the recollections of many years of masses into a few short minutes of videotaped memory, but the images that I recall most clearly are those associated with the ritual of the sign of peace—that moment in the Catholic mass when we are told to turn to our neighbor and share with him or her some sign of peace.

In my family that meant shaking hands with our siblings, with whom we were often—as siblings often are—quarreling. But no matter how serious the quarrel, no matter how irritated we were with one another entering the church, we were capable of forgiveness in that moment. The particular image that stands out in my mind from those family masses are the rueful smiles we would exchange, along with our handshakes: Wasn't I being an idiot this morning? And weren't you being one too?

The weekly ritual of mass attendance came to represent family. It was the only time during the week when all seven of us were guaranteed to be together in the same place, with none of us running in or out of the door on the way to football practice, or gymnastics, or school, or an evening out. Especially as the older siblings grew into their high school and college years, those weekly gatherings of the family became one of the few guarantees we had of seeing one another, all together.

As the sign of peace concludes, my mind drifts to thoughts of my family, and to the fact that in just a few short weeks almost all of them—with the exception of my eldest brother Tom, his wife, and their three children—will be gathering at our house for a few days after Christmas. My sister and her new husband are driving in from Chicago; my parents are doing the same from Cleveland; my youngest brother and his new wife are driving up from New York City; and my older brother Tony will be driving in with his wife and their son from New Haven.

We will be packed into our four-bedroom house, with at least one couple on the sleeper sofa in the family room, but I am certain no one will mind the crowding. Crowding is what our family has always been about, with five children and two parents growing up in a four-bedroom home in the west suburbs of Cleveland. Until Tony left for college, I never had a bedroom of my own. At one point during my childhood, after the birth of our youngest brother, I shared a bedroom with my two older brothers: two bunks crammed into one corner of the room, another bed across from it, and desks and dressers wherever we could find space for them.

I have been anticipating these few days of our holiday family reunion for months now, and can hardly stand the wait for another couple of weeks. When we are together we revert to the habits of our youth, from exchanging bone-crushing bear hugs to staying up late into the night, drinking beer and renting classic comedies— anything with Bill Murray will do (except *The Razor's Edge*, of course).

What I don't know yet, sitting in the chapel and letting my mind drift forward in anticipation, is that by the time those few days roll around I will be even sicker than I am at that moment. I will be in the bathroom as many as ten to fifteen times a day, I will be eating bland food to no avail, I will be so tired that I will occasionally have to leave the laughter and music in the family room for a short rest upstairs. I will be a source of worry and concern to all of them—but especially, again, to my mother.

What I don't know is that on the Saturday afternoon after Christmas my father will buy loads of shrimp cocktail from the store, that my little brother Billy and his wife will make their famous guacamole dip, that Tony will open a bottle of wine long before the customary cocktail hour, and that we will all gather into the family room, eating and drinking and playing with the children for several happy hours. I don't know yet that I will be too sick for any of it, that I will sit on the floor over by the stereo, changing the CDs, running back and forth to the bathroom, drinking the glass of water I have begun to carry with me everywhere to stave off the dehydration—and watching.

What I also don't know is that, over the course of those few hours, and over the course of that visit, I will begin to understand that my happiness does not necessarily have to depend upon my health. I will feel happy despite my body's best efforts to thwart me, despite the fact that I will be the only one not gorging myself on shrimp, and not drinking. Even my mother, a near teetotaler, will sip a glass of wine, her face flushed and warm.

This understanding will not undercut or alter the lessons I have been learning about the disease's influence on my mind and my emotions as well as my body. But I will begin to see that it is possible, even in the darkest moments of disease, to find solace and comfort in those parts of my life that have always provided solace and comfort to me: my family—both the one from which I have come and the one I have created with my wife and children—and my religion.

Sitting in the chapel on that early afternoon in December, I don't yet know all of this. But, in the course of that noon mass, as I follow the familiar and comfortable rituals of this religious cere- mony I have been attending for thirty years, I have begun to sense it.

We are now in the celebration of the Eucharist, and we stand—not kneeling, as we did at the church in which I grew up— and watch the priest perform the ceremonies that, according to Catholic doctrine, will turn the pieces of bread and cup of wine on the altar into the literal body and blood of Jesus Christ.

I have always felt conflicted about this doctrine of Catholicism, which requires me to suspend my belief in the laws of physics and biology in order to accept the occurrence of this miraculous trans- formation at every mass I attend. I have difficulty believing anything I cannot understand rationally, and this piece of Catholicism ranks near the top of doctrines that are rationally incomprehensible. So for most of my life I have received the Eucharist, and watched the rituals associated with it, with some dispassion.

But a few years into my struggle with the disease, while I was sitting in a mass one Sunday morning, it occurred to me that the Eucharist presented an opportunity for a sort of divine intervention in the course of my disease. It made perfect sense: Here was a piece of divinity that, instead of existing in some faraway realm of angels of heavenly bliss, actually passed through my gut! Was it pos- sible that God could use the Eucharist to soothe and heal my gut, if only I were to believe that He could do so?

The idea quickly took hold of my imagination. We were still living in Chicago then, and the disease was in a semi-active state. I could live my life, and was not experiencing any of the emotional symptoms that accompanied a serious flare, but diarrhea, the occa- sional close call, and a persistent, low-grade fatigue were all parts of my routine.

At that time we attended mass at a church that held a separate celebration, in the basement of the church, for parents with small children. It was packed with people, and with fidgety, loud children—you had no worries whatsoever that your children were disturbing anyone. In fact, you could hardly hear your own kids for the noise from other people's children.

I liked this aspect of the mass, because I have always felt that the mass should be an occasion for laughter and happiness rather than solemnity. The presence of the children necessarily made it so.

But when I began to think about the healing power of the Eucharist in my life, I began to resent all of the commotion and distraction. I wanted to pray and contemplate the Eucharistic celebration in silence, and to have a solemn atmosphere in which I could communicate to God that I really believed He could heal me.

I felt certain that this was the trick: God had obviously chosen not to heal me through the Eucharist thus far, which meant that there must still be some contribution I had to make to the process. I understood that contribution to be my complete faith in the possibility that God could heal me in this way.

I probably did not articulate this to myself at the time, but in retrospect I suspect this belief came from various biblical stories in which the belief of the sick person seems to play a crucial role in Christ's decision to heal: the story of the Roman centurion, for example, who begs Jesus to heal his sick servant, but then balks when Jesus tries to follow him to his home. "Sir," the centurion replies, "I am not worthy to have you under my roof. Just give the word and my servant will be cured." Astonished, Jesus announces to his disciples that "in no one in Israel have I found faith as great as this." The sick servant is cured.

So I needed to become that centurion, so certain that Christ had the power to heal me that He would finally consent to do so.

And I felt certain that that healing would come through the Eucharist. That little sliver of unleavened bread, I was convinced, would work its way into my colon and soothe and heal my sores in a way that conventional medicine never could.

So I prayed. And I went to mass and received the Eucharist. I did my very best to believe in its healing powers, blocking out the sounds of children all around me as I sat in church and felt it sliding into my digestive tract. I tried to envision it as a little circle of healing light, one that would illuminate the dark spaces of my colon, bearing the divine cure to me.

And—of course?—nothing happened. Did I really expect it to? I'm not sure anymore. Perhaps I never really managed to dispel my doubt that I could be healed in this way, and perhaps that sliver of doubt prevented me from receiving the sort of healing that I hoped would come from my absolute faith in Christ's powers.

My eventual abandonment of the hopes I had for such divine intervention were slow to die—so slow, in fact, that even during this December mass in the chapel I am still grasping at shards of that hope. I never made a conscious decision of any sort to reject the possibility of such healing; instead, as the Sundays stretched into months and then years, without any consistent improvement in my health, I resigned myself—or re-resigned myself, more accurately—to the idea that I could not count on God to solve my problems for me.

So as I walk slowly down the aisle to receive the Eucharist, I am reminded of my hopes for divine healing, and feel the tiniest surge of hope. Perhaps this time?

I receive the bread, place it in mouth, and say a little prayer.

But even as I do so, running beneath that prayer like a river, another part of my brain is chastising me for the falseness of it; I don't really believe it. That surge of hope is reflexive, unthinking; every other part of my brain understands that healing will not come to me in this way.

To the unbeliever, and even to some believers, this long spell of belief I had in the possibility of divine healing will seem foolish. But it is an old truth that there are no unbelievers in a foxhole; I doubt there are many unbelievers, either, among the chronically and terminally ill.

Many of those chronically ill believers look to the divine, I know from both intuition and experience, with the same hopes that I have spent the last few years struggling to overcome. They believe their deity will, out of compassion for their plight, perform a miraculous intervention in their lives and render them whole again.

But I hope that at least some of them look to the divine, and to the religions that formalize their relationships with the divine, with the understanding that has been gradually dawning on me throughout this noon mass, and that will become so important to me in the months of illness that will follow.

MY FIRST ARTICULATE SENSE of this understanding comes to me as I am back in my seat in the chapel, watching and hearing the familiar closing rituals of the mass. With a start, I realize that, for the past half hour or so, I have been happy.

I have been happy to be in a place so long associated for me with comfortable and familiar rituals. I have been happy to be in a place in which I can take the time to reflect in an unhurried manner on my life, on God, and on the relationship between the two. I have been happy to be in a place in which I feel a connection, however vague and fuzzy it might be, to a community, a world, and a spirituality larger than myself and my immediate concerns.

I have been happy to stand among flawed human beings striving to be better, all of us affirming together the importance of human community, if only for just thirty minutes on a cold December afternoon.

MASS HAS ENDED, but I am reluctant to leave. I linger in the pews, reveling in this newly articulated awareness and understanding of the role that God and religion should be playing in my life. Outside, the snow has been coming down more insistently, the wind blowing more coldly. Outside, there are papers to grade, students to see, classes to prepare for. Inside, there is peace, calm, comfort.

Over the next days and weeks, as the semester comes to a close, as I continue to anticipate the arrival of my family, and as my disease worsens, the insight that flashed upon me in the chapel that afternoon will work its way through my understanding of every part of my spiritual and religious life.

That insight will help me see the value of my God and my religion in providing me with comfort and peace even in the worst stages of my disease; it will help me see the value of the mass as providing me with familiar rituals in times when I can count on almost nothing else in my life to remain constant, from the plans I make and am forced to break to the number of times I visit the bathroom each day; it will help me understand the value of prayer as an end in itself, rather than as a means of securing favors or blessings from God.

It is this last point that has perhaps become most important to me.

The period during which I prayed for Christ to heal me

through the Eucharist, while it may have been unique in its concentration upon that one sacrament, was not out of character for me—or, I suspect, for many sufferers of chronic disease—in other ways. For most of my life, even before chronic illness, and like most people raised in religious traditions, I have been accustomed to pray in moments of crisis.

For the past half-dozen years, those moments and periods of crisis primarily have concerned my illness. Prayers for general healing, for a respite from illness in the darkest days of severe flares, and for, most simply, a handily placed public toilet in a moment of urgent need—I have let all of these prayers issue from my lips at one time or another.

And, unlike those blessed characters from the Bible with whom Christ came into contact, my prayers have almost uniformly gone unanswered. Underlying my sense that God could intervene in the course of my illness and heal me, I can see now, was the belief that God had given me Crohn's disease for some reason I could not fathom.

It has taken me almost five years to realize that God did not give me Crohn's disease—and, more importantly, that God is not going to take it away. The process of evolution, of genetics, and of environmental conditions gave me Crohn's disease. I am quite certain that God is sorry to see me suffer, and mourns with me when I mourn. But I'm also quite certain He has no plans to intervene in the course of my disease.

Does God work small miracles in people's lives—using the Eucharist, for example, to heal their digestive disorders? I don't really know. I don't know how anyone could ever know that. I hope He does, for the people who really need Him. But my disease has taught me that I cannot rely on such miracles to get me through my problems, and that my prayers are best aimed in other directions.

I pray now for the strength to fight whatever the disease can throw at me, for the wisdom that disease can bring, and for the patience to see me through to the next remission. Those are prayers that, once uttered, are already half-answered. The process of asking God for strength helps steel one for the battle; the process of asking for wisdom brings reflection and understanding; the process of asking for patience helps see one through another day.

In the movie *Shadowlands*, the character of C.S. Lewis explains at one point that he prays not to change God's mind, but to change his own. For some reason this line stuck in my head when I first heard it, many years ago, but only in the last year or so have I come to understand what it means. I pray to heal my mind, not to heal my body. And the very act of praying begins, and sometimes completes, that healing.

These spiritual insights are perhaps the most profound lessons that chronic disease has taught me. Look to what the very act of praying can do for me; don't look for answers. Go to mass to see myself as part of a community and a religion that help to place my individual problems in perspective; don't go to mass expecting miracles. Go to mass to affirm my place in this religious family.

I would be dishonest if I did not end this chapter by confessing, though, that I don't believe I can ever shut myself off completely from the possibility that answers may come, that a miracle cure for disease might be right around the corner, and that God may have a different message for me about religion and prayer.

My mother, I know, would insist that such miracle cures are entirely possible, and in fact occur quite frequently. I know she prays for such healing for me, and I know she attributes her own recovery from cancer to just such divine intervention.

But I will take, in the place of such healing, the next time she and I are able to attend mass together. The ritual of the sign of peace will come around, and she and I will exchange hugs. She will smile and look into my eyes, and she will squeeze my hand.

Such little gestures: miracles of their own.

6

THE HOSPITAL

Learning to Hit the Bottom of the Well

~

[February 2001]

I n January of 2001, my gastroenterologist finally prescribed the immunosuppressive Imuran, in the hope that the drug would help me taper off steroids and achieve a more sustained remission. But the combination of the prednisone—which also helps suppress the immune system—and the immunosuppressive left me vulnerable to infections and contagious diseases, and in mid-February I came down with a nasty stomach flu.

It happened on a Monday, just after dinner. Anne had taken the girls out shopping for something or another, and I had a quick dinner alone. Afterward I brought in some firewood from outside, intending to make us a fire for the evening. Outside it was dark, and had been since 5:00 PM, and we were in the midst of a stretch of frigid weather that had yet to dump any snow on us.

85

Before I had a chance to make the fire I began vomiting and could not stop. The disease had been more than usually active that day, and within a few hours after the vomiting had begun I was living in the bathroom, everything in my system coming out of both ends at regular intervals.

The vomiting and the diarrhea slowly worsened, and it wasn't more than five or six hours after I first became ill—between 11:00 and midnight—that I realized I was becoming dangerously dehydrated. We called a neighbor to watch the kids, my wife drove me to the hospital, and I spent the night in the emergency room, receiving IV hydration.

I wanted to be released in the morning. I didn't see that the hospital could do much for me. There is no cure for the flu, of course, and the diarrhea was the result of disease activity we all knew about. I was already taking all of the medications I could possibly take, so I didn't see the point in sticking around and losing sleep in the noisy emergency room.

They did release me, and early that morning—before 7:00—I called Anne and asked her to pick me up before she left for school. As I waited in the lobby for her, I suddenly began to feel sick again. I ran to the bathroom, where I vomited into the trash can while I sat on the toilet.

I should have turned around and walked back into the ER, but I didn't. It still seemed that the hospital had nothing to offer me.

It didn't matter much in the end. I was back in the ER the following evening, the vomiting less serious but the disease escalating out of control. When I had described the full extent of my symptoms to the nurse on call earlier that evening, she had sent an ambulance for me, so at least Anne and the girls were able to remain in bed—though I don't suppose Anne was sleeping much. I spent another night in the hospital, during which I had a very strange encounter with the nurse who had been assigned to my bed the previous evening.

THIS NURSE WAS NOT responsible for my room on that second evening, but she came in to speak with me anyway. As she talked she busied herself in the room, straightening up medical equipment, folding linen, and adjusting my bed and pillows.

She came by, she explained, because she wanted to talk to me about my illness. Her father had Crohn's disease, and for many years he had suffered as I apparently seemed to be suffering—in and out of hospitals, bouncing up and down on multiple medications, and experiencing all of the disease's unpleasant symptoms and effects.

At that point in her story I expected her to offer me the customary words of emotional support and sympathy.

It turned out, though, that she intended to offer me a more specific message.

"He finally got better," she said, referring to her father, "when he got off all of the medications they had him on and changed his diet. He went on an all-juice diet, and that cleared up his inflammation. Then he stopped taking his medications and began to eat right. He hasn't been back to the hospital since."

"Is that right?" I said.

"Listen," she told me, lowering her voice to a conspiratorial whisper. "If you keep coming back here, all they're going to do is try and put you on more and more medications. And the more medications they put you on, the more you'll come back here. It's a vicious cycle.

"They want to help you, but you don't *need* this kind of help. You need to take control of your life, take control of your diet, take control of this disease. You're the only one that can make yourself better."

She grabbed a pad of paper and wrote down several names on it.

"These are books that will help you," she said, still whispering. She thrust the paper into my hand. "These books will tell you what to eat, and how to get away from all of these medications."

She looked at me intently, still pressing the paper into the palm of my hand.

"Do you promise me that you will read these books, that you will start taking control of this disease on your own? Do you *promise me* that you will?"

I almost burst out laughing at the absurdity of it. Sitting there on the edge of my hospital bed, in her nurse's aqua-green uniform, stethoscope around the back of her neck, she was asking me to renounce everything that all of those trappings stood for. Undoubtedly she would be leaving my room to visit other patients—to administer their medications, to monitor their vital signs with expensive medical equipment, to follow the dictates of the emergency room doctors in the care of her patients.

"Sure," I said finally. "Sure. I will."

She gave my hand a squeeze and left without saying anything else.

IN THE MORNING I requested, once again, to be released. The emergency room doctor asked me if I thought I needed to be admitted. I told him I understood what was happening, and didn't see any reason for it. He agreed.

Anne was staying in regular contact with my mother, who decided to fly out and help us deal with all of the other aspects of life—like taking care of children and running a household—that

the disease was eclipsing. She brought with her everything that a
mother brings: love, compassion, help, and—especially—worry.

But she could not bring me help for my inflamed and ulcerated
gut. Even as the flu abated, the disease began to spiral out of control. By the time I was finally admitted to the hospital two days
later, I was having between twenty-five and thirty bowel movements in a twenty-four-hour period.

The nurse who greeted me when they wheeled me from the
emergency room into the room where I would stay for the next six
days asked me about this in disbelief:

"Are you the guy who was having *thirty* bowel movements a
day?"

"That's me."

"Is that *really* true?"

"I wouldn't make it up, believe me."

To discover that my symptoms were shocking even to medical
personnel certainly let me know, if my body had not yet done so
sufficiently, that I was in serious trouble.

Once I had been admitted and settled into my room, they
hooked me up to an IV machine that dispensed extremely high
doses of prednisone into my system, along with fluids to combat
the dehydration. I was in a room far at the end of the hall,
where—as one nurse kindly explained to me—I wouldn't be too
disturbed by foot traffic or other noise outside in the hall. Anne
packed the few clothes I had brought with me into the dresser
drawers the hospital provided. She sat with me for a few minutes,
but we both agreed her time was best spent at home with the girls.

Once I was alone, I began to worry immediately. Not, as one
might expect, about my health—I was worried, instead, about
school.

I had missed almost an entire week of classes, from Tuesday

through Friday, and it was clear that I would miss at least one more week. If the amount of time I had to miss were to stretch into three and four weeks, the college would be better off giving me the rest of the semester on leave, and hiring someone to take over my courses.

I did *not* want to do that, primarily because I knew we could not afford it. So I began thinking immediately about how I could have my classes covered for the following week without overtaxing any of my colleagues in the department. Assuming I would lose the next week in the hospital, I just needed to make it back for the week following that one, and then it would be spring break. I could use spring break to recover and regain my strength.

My first visitor on that first day in the hospital was the chair of my department, who absolutely assured me that the department would cover the classes until I could return, and that I should worry about nothing but my health. I wish I could have listened to that message.

Her visit simply stoked my school anxiety further. Although I should have been resting, I couldn't sleep—the prednisone, which induces sleeplessness, was at least partially responsible for that—so I plugged in my laptop and typed a long message to send around to everyone in the department, requesting their assistance. I saved the file onto a disk and later, when another friend from the department visited me, I asked him to give the disk to the department secretary and have her e-mail it to all of my colleagues.

Reprinting that message here will perhaps give the clearest picture of how I could not—despite everything that was happening to my body, mind, and family—accept the idea that the world would go on spinning without me:

Dear Colleagues:
First of all, thanks to all of you for the flowers, and to many of you for your individual expressions of concern and offers to

help. And especially thanks to Mike Land for helping me coordi-
nate all of this, and thanks in advance to any of you who can
respond to this call for assistance. . . .

I canceled classes last week from Tuesday through Friday,
but this week would like to try and have most of my classes meet
if that will be possible. The great news is that I had planned this
week to have almost no preparation, because I needed to write
a conference paper this week! I have canceled that conference,
so that means I can relax this week. To add to the good fortune,
my mother has come from Florida to help out around the
house, and my wife has off next week because of school vacation. So she can help do some of the leg work for this stuff.
Having my Mom here is a weird kind of irony, because this place
reminds me of Florida, when we visit my parents on spring
break—lots of old people, not much to do besides read and
relax. Of course the beach and restaurants would be nice, but
you can't have everything.

At any rate, you will see from below that in almost all of the
classes I have to teach this week, with one exception, absolutely
no preparation is required at all. What I hoped to do was lay
out the dates and times for all of my classes, and if you are able
to perform some very minimal duties you can let Mike know
and then just give me a quick call at the hospital if you have any
questions. My number here in this palatial suite is 363-8649. I
am pumped up on IV steroids so I am ALWAYS awake. So here
goes. . . .

The message went on to describe what I was doing in each of
my classes, with detailed instructions for my substitutes.

Despite the good humor I mustered in parts of the message,
the emotion that animated these instructions was panic. When I
had been sick in August, it had been prior to the start of school,
and the lack of defined and immediate tasks had allowed me to slip
into that state of apathy and depression that lasted me into the

beginning of the school year. I wasn't getting anything done then, but it didn't really matter.

This time around, I had a schedule—courses to teach, meetings to attend, students to advise, and writing deadlines to meet. Moreover, at our college we teach on a 3–4 schedule, which means we have three classes during one semester and four the next. The spring semester was my four-course semester, increasing my duties by 25 percent. Finally, the rapidity and severity with which the disease had overtaken me this time meant that I did not have weeks or months to spend slowly sinking into the usual state of apathy or depression that accompanies a longer flare. When I entered the hospital I was still in the mental and emotional state that usually lasts me through the first days and weeks of a flare—trying to fight off the disease, to postpone the inevitable by exercising more regularly, watching my diet more closely, and getting extra sleep.

This mode always carries with it a great deal of anxiety and frustration, because such homeopathic therapies never work. If I have reached the stage at which I am aware that a flare is coming on quickly, then I am usually too far gone to help myself without more conventional medicines.

This mind-set—the attitude that I can fight off the disease, and will not let it interrupt my life—is probably more responsible than any of my other behaviors for the severity of some of the flares I have experienced. It has led to the postponement of regular medicinal interventions, to higher levels of anxiety and stress, and to a divided mental state in which I am desperately trying to ward off the disease on the one hand, and increasingly frustrated, on the other hand, at the ineffectiveness of my efforts.

More than anything else, the hospital helped me to see the futility of this attitude and the toll on emotional, physical, and psychological energy that comes with it. My stay in the hospital helped me learn how to hit bottom and let go—to learn when to surrender myself to the therapies and medications that will help me recover from a flare most effectively and most quickly, and to let modern medicine do its work.

That sort of letting go does not mean abandoning control of my medical care—as I will explain shortly, my continued monitoring and input on that care remained essential. But it does mean that, when I have really hit bottom, I cannot expect my body to heal itself miraculously, or to respond quickly and easily to the sorts of suggestions that the nurse had given me on that second night in the emergency room: all-juice diets, or radical dietary prescriptions of any sort.

I remain hopeful that those sorts of remedies might one day be effective for me in maintaining remission, or in managing moderate disease activity. But when I am lying at the bottom of the well, the recommendations of that nurse are a siren's song: They tempt and tease me with the belief that I can take control of my disease and heal myself.

Letting go, by contrast, means acknowledging that the disease has temporarily taken control of my life, and that I need help to regain that control. Letting go means accepting that help willingly and gratefully.

MY SIX DAYS in the hospital settled quickly into routine. Of course, routines come easily enough when you have an IV line attached to your arm and can't venture more than fifty feet from a restroom.

Someone usually woke me up around 6:30 or 7:00 AM to check my vital signs and give me some medication. After that initial wakeup, I would lie in bed for another hour, drifting in and out of sleep until breakfast.

When breakfast was finished at 8:30 or so, I read until mid-morning, when I usually tried to sleep a little. After lunch I did the same thing. Read for a couple of hours, and sleep for a couple of hours.

Anne usually arrived around or shortly after dinnertime, and we would sit together and read our books or watch television. Sometimes we lay together in my hospital bed; sometimes I would let her lie in the hospital bed and I would sit in the chair in my room, just for a change.

Usually Anne came alone. She had brought Katie and Madeleine on my first evening in the hospital, but it was quickly apparent to both of us that my hospital room was not very child-friendly. After fifteen minutes of hugging, playing with the controls on my hospital bed, and peering out at the hallway traffic, they were ready to go. We agreed, after that initial visit, that Anne would leave the children with my mother in the future.

Anne usually stayed until nine o'clock or even ten on some evenings, and when she left I watched another hour of television or read. The night nurse came around 10:00 with my final medications for the day, including sleeping pills. I took those at 11:00, and was usually out for the night by 11:30.

All of this was punctuated by regular trips to the restroom, though the daily number of those trips began gradually to decrease: from twenty-five or thirty to twenty, to fifteen, and down to eight or ten by the time I was ready to leave.

As the week passed, I began slowly to loosen my hold on the world, and to learn to let go in a second way: to relax my desperate grip on those parts of my life that would survive, at least temporarily, without me.

What I needed was simply to rest. I had initially asked Anne to bring my laptop and all of my schoolwork to my room, so that I could read ahead for when I returned. She also brought me, though, Arthur Golden's *Memoirs of a Geisha*, a novel she had recently read and loved. For the first day or two I worked half-heartedly at my schoolwork. By Monday I had abandoned it and was spending all of my time reading—and enjoying immensely—Golden's novel.

I had a massive stack of papers to grade; they sat ungraded in my schoolbag in the closet. I had lots of phone calls I wanted to make, to friends and even family members with whom I had not spoken in some time; I enjoyed the quiet and silence of my room. As usual, I had essays and children's books and novel ideas floating around in my head, waiting to be put down on paper; my laptop remained in its carrying case in the corner of the room.

The farther along in the week I got, the more I began to sleep and relax, and slowly, almost infinitesimally at first, I could feel my body beginning to heal.

IN THE HOSPITAL I did discover one area where I could not relax my guard, however.

I had initially brought all of my medications to the hospital with me when we came for the third and final time. The nurses let me know immediately, though, that the hospital would take control of my medication schedule while I was in their care, including both providing my pills and bringing them to me at the appropriate times.

This worked fine until my third day.

As always, I had one medication I was supposed to take at around 2:00 PM. This was also usually the time that the nurses changed shifts. The afternoon nurse generally would come in to see me with my medications and introduce herself sometime between 2:00 and 2:30.

On that third day, I had slept for a while after lunch, and woke up to begin reading around 1:30. I had one eye on the clock, waiting for my early afternoon medication. When you have so little to do and think about, each visit from the nurses becomes a marker in the passing day. Two o'clock passed without a visit, as did 2:30 and 3:00. I continued to read halfheartedly, expecting a nurse to come swirling in at any moment, in a rush from some emergency in another part of the hospital, apologizing for her lateness.

By four o'clock I suspected that someone had overlooked me, and I buzzed for a nurse.

"Hello," she said brightly as she entered my room, a few moments later. "Did you buzz?"

"Ahhhhh . . . In the past, they had been giving me my Asacol at 2:00 PM, but I didn't get any today. Did they change my schedule?" I didn't want to accuse her directly of neglect.

"Oh," she said, genuinely perplexed. "Hold on a second."

She returned five minutes later with a chart in her hand, and a small cup with my pills in it. "I'm sorry," she said. "Somehow we got this mixed up."

Of course human error occurs in every profession, and of course this particular mistake was quickly rectified and, in the big picture, probably would not have made any difference in the course of my healing. But it was disconcerting for me to see it happen, and to be reminded that human error was as likely to occur in a profession in which people's health and lives were at stake as it was in any other profession.

I suppose I should have been prepared for something like that to happen, had I thought more about the food they were serving me.

The doctor who saw me on my first full day had suggested to me, in a general conversation about my health and diet, that I avoid lactose for a while. Lactose is difficult to digest, and so—even if I were not lactose-intolerant—it would make sense for me to keep it out of my diet until I had settled down.

On my very next meal tray, I received a carton of milk.

I left it untouched, thinking that perhaps the doctor's orders had not reached the food service people yet. At the next meal, and every meal thereafter, a carton of milk showed up on my tray.

For the first few days I was there, they kept me on a liquid diet of broth, Jell-O, juice, and water. When they finally switched me off that diet, I was expecting to receive softened and easily digestible foods like rice, pasta, and whipped potatoes. Instead, the first tray of regular food I received included a cup of raw fruit, green beans, and chicken.

I had enough experience with dietitians to know that raw fruits and vegetables were probably the worst substances I could put into my body at that point. Sending fruits and vegetables into my damaged colon was, as one dietitian colorfully described it to me, like running a whisk broom over an open sore.

I picked away at the pasta side dish, drank the juice, and ate a few pieces of chicken. It was not the sort of first solid meal I had been expecting.

After a day or two more of this I began to get a little card with the daily menus on it, and I could select my own foods. I wondered if anyone was monitoring that. If I selected bran flakes and milk, fruit, and raw broccoli for every meal, would they bring it to me? In retrospect, it seems highly doubtful that anyone would have said anything.

Eventually I said something to the nurse and they switched my thrice-daily carton of milk to one of Lactaid, a lactose-free milk that tastes virtually the same as milk.

I had one final experience with the doctors in the hospital that reaffirmed the commitment I had made earlier that year to becoming my own best patient advocate.

The first physician who saw me was a general practitioner, a young man with a friendly bedside manner who apparently did the rounds covering my ward.

He, to the best of my understanding, ordered my dose of IV medication and controlled and monitored any other treatment I was to receive.

On my first day in the hospital he laid out a general plan of treatment for me. I would remain on the IV steroids for a day or two, and would then begin taking oral steroids at a dose of 80 milligrams per day—double the highest dose I had ever taken before. I would remain at that dose until I had settled down, and then I would begin tapering down the dose. He was not sure how long I would stay in the hospital.

Then he said something that surprised me.

"We will probably take you off the Imuran, since that could be causing the vomiting."

"I thought the flu was causing the vomiting," I said.

"It may be. This would be more of a precautionary measure. I'll check with your GI before I order any changes, but I suspect that's what he'll tell me."

I was upset by this. I had been taking the Imuran for five weeks or so, and had been initially told by my gastroenterologist—and had confirmed this with my own research—that it could take as long as four to twelve weeks to begin having any effect on the body. If I stopped it now, did that mean I would have to start the cycle all over again, and potentially wait another twelve weeks before I could really begin to see its positive effects?

I kept my mouth shut for the moment, figuring that I would

fight that battle if and when they actually stopped giving me the Imuran.

My gastroenterologist, by an unlucky coincidence, had been on vacation in Hawaii for three weeks when this began, so he didn't visit me until my fifth day in the hospital. Instead, colleagues from his group practice came and saw me to monitor my condition.

On the same day I had spoken with the first doctor, one of his colleagues came in with two residents and gave me a brief examination. He was a young and handsome doctor, the sort you might expect to see on a television soap opera, and his residents were even younger.

The trio sat on the bed opposite me and the doctor began to ask me questions.

"How long has this been going on?" he said.

I thought I could hear an implied criticism in there—how could anyone possibly let themselves get this out of control?—but I could have been imagining it. I reacted to it anyway.

"A long time," I said. "I guess I knew I should have done something, but I was waiting for the Imuran to kick in, and I knew it could take four to twelve weeks, and it's been five weeks now. I was hoping that would begin to settle me down."

"Imuran," he said to me, without even looking up from my chart, "can take three to six *months* to begin working."

Upon hearing that, my heart just sank. I could have another five months of this? I was also embarrassed—he said it in a way that implied anyone should have known *that*. I thought I saw the two residents glance at one another, a silent smirk—stupid patients.

"Really?"

"Yes. You can't really wait, at this stage, for Imuran to begin solving the problem. In fact, we need to evaluate whether Imuran is causing your current problems with nausea."

"I thought that was from the flu."

"Well," he said, "that's possible—but that's why we're here, so we can tell you for certain. I'll talk to your regular GI when he returns tomorrow."

The three of them left abruptly. The exchange had lasted no more than three minutes, and I had never felt stupider and more doubtful of my ability to gain credible knowledge about my medical treatment.

For the next two days I continued to receive the Imuran, so I assumed that both physicians were waiting to let my regular gastroenterologist make the final decision.

But two days later a third gastroenterologist, another colleague of my regular physician, came to see me. I learned from him that my regular physician was back in the office and would visit the next day.

In the meantime, this third doctor's recommendation was that I receive injections of a growth hormone that had proved useful in controlling severe inflammations of the disease. Those injections, a relatively new treatment, would perhaps see me through to when the Imuran would begin to take effect. He would not order them for me, but would recommend them to my physician.

"And will I keep taking the Imuran?" I said to him as he was leaving.

"Of course," he said.

Finally, my own gastrotenterologist returned and came to see me on the day before I left. We exchanged greetings and he asked me some questions about my bowel habits in the last few days.

"I must admit," he said to me after these exchanges, "that I was a bit disconcerted to hear that you were here when I got back. I was expecting things to improve for you after we had started you on the Imuran."

"Me too."

"I found that a little disconcerting," he repeated. He seemed disconcerted. "But it looks to me like you are beginning to heal. I suspect we will let you go home tomorrow, and you can continue the steroid treatments until you are more fully under control."

"Will I keep taking the Imuran?"

"Yes. We'll continue with all of your current medications."

"One of the doctors who saw me recommended some kind of hormone injections. Are we going to do anything like that?"

"I don't think that will be necessary, as long as you are showing signs of improvement."

We spoke for a bit longer about my treatment, he instructed me to set up a follow-up appointment, and we said good-bye.

In the six days I had spent in the hospital, I had seen four doctors and been recommended three different courses of treatment. I had learned my lesson about doctors and medicine in September, in my dealings with the university physicians, but this incident reminded me that such lessons cannot be packed away and confined to my dealings with any particular physician. The uncertainties of diagnosis and therapy will follow me through this disease, and in those areas—and possibly only those areas—however close I am to the bottom, I can never let go.

HAVING TOLD A NUMBER of stories about my interactions with physicians that cast them in a fairly unforgiving light, I must finish this chapter with the story of the one physician who deserves to be named in this narrative, and who has helped to maintain my faith in the medical establishment.

To do that, I need to circle back to the beginning of this chapter.

After the two consecutive nights upon which I had been admitted to the emergency room, only to return home the following day, I received a telephone call from my internist, Dr. Robert Honig.

I had always been happy with Dr. Honig as a physician, and enjoyed my visits to him. He was never a minute late for an appointment, despite his evident interest in the details of our lives—he was always interested in discussing the academic life with me, and always wanted to know about whatever book I had brought in with me to read—and despite his willingness to pay serious attention to whatever medical complaint one brought to him. He explained any treatment he ordered in comprehensive detail, but in terms I could understand. He was the internist for a number of us at the college, and all of us had stories testifying to his unusually personable and attentive treatment of his patients.

"How you doing, Professor?" he asked me, when he called me that morning.

I explained what I had been going through the last couple of days, and we agreed that I would let him know if I saw no signs of improvement within the next day or two, or any changes for the worse.

The next morning my mother, my wife, and I all decided that we could not continue dealing with this level of disease activity on our own. We called Dr. Honig and let him know we thought it was time for me to return to the hospital.

It was a Saturday morning. I telephoned the call line—his office was closed on Saturdays—and he returned my call within ten minutes.

"Go to the hospital now," he said. "I'll meet you in the emergency room. We'll get you in faster that way."

In the emergency room a nurse checked my insurance information, and then instructed me to wait until an admitting desk was free. We sat down; a few minutes later, Dr. Honig came in and greeted us, shaking my hand as he always did.

"Let me see if I can speed this process up," he said.

He went over to the admitting desks and spoke to someone there for a moment. Then he waved us over, and stood behind us while they took additional information from us. The admitting clerk told us that I would still need to wait for a hospital bed, but that they would get me into one as quickly as possible.

Dr. Honig disappeared behind the administrative doors of the emergency room, and was back shortly to let me know that some beds were opening up, and I would be taken upstairs soon. Sure enough, ten minutes later I was on a mobile bed, IV in my arm, waiting for an orderly to transport me upstairs.

Dr. Honig promised to return in a few days.

On my third day there he walked through the door of my room late one afternoon with a smile on his face and his usual greeting:

"How ya' doing, Professor?"

"I'm getting there."

"It sucks, doesn't it?"

He sat down in the chair next to my bed and spent a few minutes commiserating with me. He wanted to know how I was handling the time I was missing at school, and how my wife and children were holding up. I was half waiting for him to begin his examination, and give me some news about my treatment, but he never did either of those things.

After he left, I realized he had never examined me. He had spoken to me about my treatment only because he seemed curious to know what I had been told by the attending physicians and gastroenterologists. The moment I understood this was the moment I realized that he had been visiting me only in part as my physician—he had also been coming to visit me as a friend. I was a human being to him, not a disease process.

As I reflected afterward upon his treatment of me throughout this period, it occurred to me that he, too, had been letting go to a certain extent—to the same extent, actually, that I had needed to let go.

He did not abdicate his care of me. He confirmed my decision to enter the hospital, he saw me through the doors of the emergency room and into a hospital bed. And I have no doubt that he checked my charts to monitor my treatment.

But he recognized, too, that my disease had proceeded beyond the point at which he—as an internist—could help me medically, and that my treatment belonged in the hands of the specialists who had greater familiarity with my disease.

From him I learned the value of the physician who knows how to let go. I have dealt with at least four different internists since I have had my disease, and have watched them attempt to assert different levels of control over my medical care. While I don't want an internist who sends me running to a specialist for every twinge and stab of pain I feel, I do want someone who recognizes when my care needs to move to the next level of specialization.

Observing his care of me, and seeing his actions and attitude parallel the one I was developing during that period, reaffirmed for me what I learned over the two weeks I spent in and out of the hospital: When you are at the bottom of the well, you need someone who knows the contours of that well to throw you a rope. It remains my responsibility to grab the rope when it comes, but I will always be the first to know I am down there.

I need to send up that cry for help, and to trust that the rope will come.

7

THE IMAGINATION
OF DISEASE

Learning to Be a Father

[February–April 2001]

One unfortunate consequence of my hospitalization was that it brought a temporary halt to our efforts to conceive a third child. Anne and I had been making halfhearted efforts toward that goal until that point. The "half" part of halfhearted came from me—Anne was far more enthusiastic about the possibility of this third child than I was.

I felt I had good reason to be halfhearted. Crohn's disease has a clear genetic component; 20 percent of sufferers have a relative who has the disease as well. The disease did not manifest itself in me until I was in my early twenties, and in that respect I was lucky. It can strike children as young as three or four years old. For those unfortunates, childhood can be a painful experience, physically and emotionally. Place yourself in the skin of a child who has to rush from the classroom frequently for trips to the restroom, who might miss weeks or months of school to illness, who might suffer excessive acne, facial bloating, and even stunted growth as a result of his or her medications.

As any parent will easily imagine, one of the most emotionally disturbing visions of my future now centers upon the prospect of seeing my children suffer from this disease. To envision any of my children undergoing what I have experienced this past year is so acutely painful to me that I wince at the thought of it.

As much as she empathizes with my condition, Anne simply will never be able to understand this fully. She has not experienced the disease as I have, and she will not be the one whose faulty genetic code may lead one of our children to a life of disease. Of course it would be irrational to see myself as somehow blameworthy if one of my children should inherit the disease, but I am afraid those feelings would overwhelm me all the same.

So while part of me shared Anne's desire for a third child, part of me resisted. My stay in the hospital strengthened the case for both of these parts: Seeing the bottom of the well increased my anxiety about the possibility of a child suffering that same fate; spending time away from my children helped me remember how much they meant to me, and sparked a desire to continue to see our family grow.

In the weeks immediately following my stay in the hospital, I felt no pressure to make any concrete decisions about whether or not we should redouble our efforts to conceive another child. I barely had enough energy to get my body up the stairs, much less spend time in bed with Anne.

I had another, far more immediate concern to worry about in those two weeks: the two children we already had.

FOR GOOD OR ILL, a combination of circumstances prevented me from understanding the effects of my hospitalization—and my illness in general—upon Katie and Madeleine until I had been home from the hospital for at least a week. When that understanding finally came, it was as devastating to my emotional stability as the illness had been to my physical health.

While I had been in the hospital, Anne had continued to teach full time, and, with the help of my mother, to pack Katie off to kindergarten and Madeleine to daycare every day by herself—not to mention cooking, taking care of the house, and worrying about me.

We had kept the girls away from the hospital because of the lack of entertainment for them there, and I suppose from an unstated agreement that they were not yet ready to face this part of my life.

When I did return home from the hospital, on a Thursday morning in late February, I was extremely weak and fatigued, and had trouble making it up and down the stairs more than a few times a day. Lying in a hospital bed for six days, along with the effects of the disease, had robbed me of most of my strength and energy. I had four days to recover before I had to be back in the classroom for one week until the semester's spring break. When spring break came I would be able to rest and recover at a more leisurely pace.

Hence I was not much of a playmate for the girls for those first few days, and beyond that for the first few weeks, after I returned home. While they began to venture outside to play, in the slowly warming weather of a New England spring, I couldn't do much more than pull up a chair on the back deck, huddled in my jacket, and watch them. Moreover, I had fallen so far behind at school that I had to reserve any energy I could muster for catching up on my grading and class preparations.

Through all of this, I had been happy to see that neither of the children ever seemed very strongly affected by my illness. When they visited me that one time in the hospital and when I watched them from the couch in our family room, they continued to do the sorts of things that small children always do: play with one another, play by themselves, fight over toys, demand snacks and juice, and pop over to give me the occasional hug and kiss. But they did not seem to me especially concerned about what was happening to me—or at least they never expressed such concerns to me or Anne.

I was quite content with this. I did not need my children feeling sorry for me and worrying about me—I had enough family members and friends already doing that. The last thing I wanted at that time was the additional burden of thinking that I was causing them psychological distress. I was happy to see them continuing with their lives as if nothing unusual were happening.

I have learned throughout my eight years or so as a parent that children can be extremely perceptive, and that even the smallest anxieties can weigh heavily on their minds. I am not sure, then, why I allowed myself to be so blind to how my hospitalization was affecting my children, my older daughter in particular. I suppose perhaps I needed that blindness; at that time I had just enough psychological energy to maintain my own balance and had none to spare for the rest of my family.

I had one early warning sign of what was happening to Katie just a few days after I returned home from the hospital. On Monday she came home with a picture from school that depicted my return from the hospital, with our family all together again. I asked her why she drew that particular scene, and she responded:

"We were supposed to draw the happiest day we could remember."

That drawing made me suddenly aware that, contrary to what

I had imagined, Katie had really been aware of my absence from home. Neither my wife nor my mother had reported to me that the girls had been excessively mournful during that absence, so I had assumed that—while I knew they loved me and missed me—they had been able to fill that gap with the excitement of having their grandmother in town.

And that may have been partially true. But my absence had made more of an impact on Katie than I had suspected.

The full extent of that impact did not become clear until several weeks later, when my wife ran into Katie's teacher at a conference. She learned then that, during the week I spent in the hospital, Katie had been upset and anxious at school, complaining of stomach pains, and had even cried on one occasion—something she rarely did in class.

The Monday after I came home from the hospital, she complained to her teacher that she had a stomachache, and asked if she could be sent home. Her teacher knew that I was recuperating from an illness, and decided that it would be better if she could find a way to keep her at school. She pressed her about how she felt, at which point Katie admitted that she did not have a stomachache at all, but wanted to be sent home so she could spend time with me.

"I miss my daddy," she told her teacher, beginning to cry.

When my wife reported this to me—and I could not hold back a few tears myself—it was like hearing a piece of bad news which, somewhere deep down, you knew was coming.

Over the next several days, I tried to involve Katie in a conversation about how she had felt when I was away, in the hope that I could perhaps relieve any lingering anxieties. I repeated to her what her teacher had told me, and asked her if it were true that she had been upset and crying at school.

"Yes," she said simply. "I missed you."

But she wouldn't elaborate any more than that, despite her normal tendency to chatter on endlessly about everything in the world. I suspected that forcing her to remember and think about the whole incident was causing her additional distress, so I stopped speaking with her about it—though that didn't stop me, of course, from worrying about it.

MADELEINE'S RESPONSE to this situation, in the meantime, could not have been more different; her contrasting reaction undoubtedly stemmed from her own particular stages of emotional and intellectual development.

Madeleine has always preferred her mother to me. My guess is that this is because Anne spent more time at home with Madeleine after her birth—over four months—than she did with Katie. Moreover, I spent one or two days a week at home with Katie when she was an infant; after Madeleine's birth, I was working full time. These are my speculations, but who really knows?

My stay in the hospital entrenched Madeleine deeper in her patterns of affection. When I finally began to spend time with the children again, it was apparent that Madeleine had grown unused to me.

In my interactions with her, I felt more like the uncle who occasionally visits from afar than the father who lives with her: the sort of adult figure who inspires a distant—because obliged—affection, some fear, and uncertainty.

Consider a typical morning, in late March, two weeks after I had returned to school from my spring break, and nearly five weeks after my stay in the hospital. As usual, Anne awakes before I do to prepare herself for the day. The girls wake up when she does, and so she sends them downstairs to watch television until one of us comes down to make their breakfast.

I pull myself groggily out of bed when Anne begins drying her hair, at which point sleep—thanks to the noise of the hair dryer—is no longer possible. I stumble downstairs and, over the protests of the girls, switch off the television in the family room.

"You can watch it while you eat your breakfast," I say. "Come into the kitchen."

I turn on the small television on the kitchen counter—the girls settle immediately into their chairs at the kitchen table, mesmerized again by the glowing screen—and pull together some breakfast foods: a bowl of Cheerios and a half of a banana for each of them.

Katie begins to eat as I set the food in front of her, but I have to tap Madeleine on the head and point out that her breakfast awaits. She turns her full attention away from the television and looks at the breakfast I have made. Her mouth sets.

"I don't want that," she says quietly.

"Madeleine," I sigh, hopeful that I can reason with her, "you *like* Cheerios and bananas. What's wrong with this breakfast?"

"I don't want that," she repeats.

I react quickly. Stupidly.

"Fine," I say, "then you don't get anything. You can starve."

She won't look at me.

"I want Mama to make it."

I knew that was coming, and it frustrates me. Of course I should react with patience and understanding—but it's 7:30 AM and I don't have the time for this and I want to be helpful to my wife, to let her experience a few moments this morning when she will not have to make breakfasts or dress her children, when she might be able to sit and have some coffee and some cereal. For the past six weeks I have been almost completely useless around the house, and now that my strength and energy are returning I want to begin to carry my load again. Madeleine is not letting me do that.

"Mama is busy; she's drying her hair. Mama doesn't have time to do everything for you. *I* can make your breakfast. *I* can help you out. *I* love you, too, you know."

My words come out angrily, not how I want them to sound, even though I am indeed feeling anger. I want to sound patient, reasonable, understanding. Katie picks up the tone in my voice, and she is watching now, paying attention to my words and to Madeleine's reaction.

Madeleine's lower lip begins to quiver. "I want Mama to make it."

I can hear the hair dryer stop upstairs, which means that Anne will be down in a minute or two. Do I fight this battle?

"She always has to have Mama, Dad," Katie says to me sympathetically.

And if I always let her have Mama, will she ever change? Do I force her to let me help her, giving her no choice in the matter— *eat what I serve or eat nothing*—so that she gets used to the idea? Or will the use of such ultimatums simply turn her against me even further? Do I simply wait for her to come to me for help on her own?

But what if she never comes?

I am standing at the counter contemplating these questions, watching Madeleine stare steadfastly into her unwanted bowl of Cheerios, unwilling even to look at me. I can hear Anne coming down the stairs, and I am still meditating on how to react when nature intervenes with its usual demand and I step quickly into the bathroom. By the time I get out Madeleine is munching happily on a piece of toast that Anne has made for her. The half of a banana and full bowl of Cheerios are sitting, untouched, on the counter.

When the time comes to get them dressed, we don't have the luxury of pondering the subtleties of the appropriate parenting strategy: I dress Katie, and Anne dresses Madeleine.

Anne is leaving before me this morning, so I help gather together backpacks and lunches and bundle everyone toward the door. I snatch a quick hug from Katie, and plant myself in front of Madeleine as she scurries to follow Anne out the door, trying to attach herself to Anne's pant leg.

"Can I have a hug?" I say.

She pushes her body around my leg, trying to worm her way out. I reach down and give her a crushing bear hug. "I love you anyway, Madeleine," I say, and kiss her on the cheek.

She smiles just a little bit—just enough so that I know I still have a chance—and then she is out the door and down the walk, chasing after Anne, calling "Mama! Mama!"

This behavior continues, it seems to me, for weeks and weeks. And for weeks and weeks I am frustrated, angry, depressed, and baffled by it. I don't really know how to react, and Anne doesn't either.

I am saved, in the end, by what Madeleine calls our "projecks."

IT IS A LATE APRIL DAY, a Wednesday afternoon, and the weather seems like it is just about ready to begin behaving as if it were spring. Green buds and shoots are making their appearance in the bushes and trees around the neighborhood, and the temperatures have been climbing consistently enough that we have confidently put away our winter jackets.

I have picked up Katie from school at 2:25. Together we drive to pick up Madeleine from her in-home daycare provider, and we are home by 2:45. Katie wants desperately to play with a neighbor girl her age, so I arrange that quickly and Madeleine and I walk her down the street to her friend's house.

Back at home I am tempted to turn on the television and lie on the couch—it has been a long semester, and I am often still tired—but for the past few weeks I have had something in mind for Madeleine, and this seems like the most opportune time.

We had brought back a box of shells from our recent vacation in Florida at my parents' condominium two weeks ago, and I have been promising her that we will do one of our projects with the shells.

"Get your box of shells, Madeleine," I tell her.

"Are we going to do a projeck, Dad?" she asks me. Her eyes are wide with anticipation.

"Get the shells, kiddo."

She goes dashing off to find the shells, and I find the large poster board I have bought in anticipation of this event. I spread it out on the dining room table with some construction paper, a tube of glue, scissors, and a box of crayons. I begin cutting out fish shapes from the construction paper, drawing little smiles and eyes on them in profile.

Madeleine returns with the box of shells, and we settle down side by side at the table.

"What are you cutting, Dad? What are *those*, Dad? Are they *fish*? Can I *help* you do that, Dad?" She says it with such a sense of enthusiasm and anticipation that I can't help but smile.

"We're going to make a beach project today, Madeleine. Let's color in the sand and the water, and then we'll glue on the shells and the fish."

"I can do it! I can do it!"

She is almost desperate with anticipation, bouncing up and down in her seat. She doesn't even know what it is she is claiming she can do; she just knows that whatever we're doing, she wants to be involved.

"Okay, kiddo," I say. "Settle down. We'll do it together."

I draw a beige line across the middle of the poster, and then give her the crayon.

"Color in the sand, all below this line," I tell her.

She begins scribbling furiously, covering the poster in long strokes of sandy crayon. I have to keep pointing out the places she has left white. We repeat the same process for the water and the sky. As she colors I continue to cut out more shapes: an octopus, a dolphin, a starfish, a sea turtle.

Finally we arrive at the moment she has been waiting for: the gluing. She is obsessed with gluing things together.

"Not too much glue now," I tell her, though I know the warning is futile.

She holds the tube of glue over the back side of a fish, a look of determination in her eyes, her little hands squeezing with all their might. The glue comes squirting out, too much; at just under three, she does not yet have the rational capacity to understand that she must stop squeezing *before* the required amount of glue actually hits the paper. The glue coats the entire back of the fish, thickly.

"Madeleine!" I say, too loud, wiping off the excess with a paper towel. "Just a little bit of glue!"

"Sorry, Daddy," but not really meaning it, breathless with anticipation at the prospect of gluing another fish. I have to remind her that, once she has applied the glue, she actually needs to paste the fish into our colored ocean.

And so we work through the project, slowly, Madeleine gluing everything she can get her hands on, me occasionally losing my temper at the mess she creates but mostly enjoying myself. For the shells I fill a Dixie cup with glue and we use toothpicks to dab it along the edges of the shells. We scatter them around the beach, scallop and mussel and clam shells and sand dollars. When we are finished I take a brown marker and carefully etch into one corner our signature project line: "Madeleine and Daddy 4/19/01."

She is immensely proud of it and wants to hang it immediately on the wall downstairs, where the children's artworks provide the decorations for the finished portion of our basement. I have to convince her to wait, explaining to her for the hundredth time how glue has to dry.

Over the next few months Madeleine and I will do project after project, most of them involving gluing something onto something else: I draw a picture of a tree, we collect leaves and acorns and glue them onto the picture; I cut out the shape of a butterfly and we glue scraps of paper to its wings; I collect shiny objects and we glue them to paper plates to make alien spacecrafts.

And over the next few months, I gradually work my way back into Madeleine's affection, gluing together a relationship that I once feared had been irremediably splintered by my illness. The rebuilding of my relationship with her reminded me so much of gluing that it was uncanny—only this time, I was the one who needed help understanding how to apply the glue properly.

In the mending of our love, I wanted to take the glue and dump it all in at once, hoping that I could resolve everything quickly. Madeleine forced me to glue properly: to apply the glue slowly, in small dabs, and to be patient and wait for the first drops to dry before applying the next ones. With each project I dabbed another drop into the crack, and with each of those drops the crack sealed a little further, and held a little more firmly.

Madeleine and I are friends now. She still has a special relationship with Anne, and no doubt she always will, but she and I have our own special kind of relationship. I am back in her life, and—at least for the moment—she believes that I'm here to stay.

THE FIX FOR KATIE was nowhere near as simple as this. The difference between two or three years old and five years old is significant, and I couldn't paper over the memories of my hospital stay in her mind with some glue and construction paper. At the moment I am writing this sentence, over a year after hitting bottom, I am quite certain that Madeleine—now four—has no recollection of my stay in the hospital; I am equally certain that Katie does.

Initially, all I could provide for Katie was my presence, both emotional and physical. I simply had to be there with her as much as possible in order to dispel the anxiety that I would go away again. I understood how important that presence was to her one afternoon in the late spring when I had picked her up from school.

At her school the parents wait for their children outside a chain-link fence that encloses the playground, and a couple dozen of us—mostly the parents of kindergartners and first- or second-graders—gather there every afternoon to wait for the bells that send our children out to us.

Many of the parents, almost all mothers, know one another. As I stand at the fence I listen to them talk about their children, about neighborhood gossip, or about the weather. I mostly keep to myself; I know one or two of them, but I am content to stand alone and watch for the kids to spill from the front doors, laughter and bundled energy bursting in little streams from the school.

On this particular afternoon, a happily warm and sunny one, Katie spies me immediately and smiles, walking quickly over to where I stand waiting. As soon as she reaches me outside the fence, she slips her hand in mine and pulls me down the sidewalk toward home. For some reason I take note of her action, and become especially conscious of the warmth of her small hand in mine.

It's a ten-minute walk home, and holding hands with a smallish

five-year old, when you are weaving your way through hordes of
children and teenagers coming from school, can be a difficult trick.
About halfway home, caught in the middle of a group of jostling
middle-schoolers, I drop her hand.

For a minute or so, we continue whatever conversation we are
having without interruption. And then, without a word or a pause
in her step, she reaches up again and grabs my hand. We hold
hands the rest of the way home.

That second grab of my hand catches my attention, and I begin
to notice that, in the weeks and months following my hospitalization, holding hands becomes a habit for us. It clearly offers her a
reassurance that she needs, and I am glad to make it available to
her.

But, of course, I won't be around to hold her hand all the time.
At some much later point, too, I know she won't want to hold my
hand anymore. The reassurance of my presence provides her with
some relief, but I can see clearly that it is a temporary solution.

It is a temporary solution for me as well.

Chronic disease induces hypochondria not only for my own
health, but also for the health of my children. All parents worry
about their children's welfare, and I am no different. But I have
the added concern—as do many parents with genetic disorders or
diseases of any sort—that my children are especially vulnerable to
my specific condition.

Every time a child complains to me of a stomachache, or diarrhea, or excessive gas, or of an urgent need to use the restroom,
my radar goes up. Until I see a complete return to normalcy, that
complaint lodges itself into my brain and tugs at the strings of my
paranoia and hypochondria. Once, on vacation in St. Louis, I
thought I saw a reddish streak in Madeleine's bowel movement;
when we returned home I immediately took her to the doctor, who

could find nothing wrong. When Katie was four years old she spent the spring complaining of stomachaches. Anne assured me that this was the commonest of childhood complaints, and likely meant nothing. I wasn't satisfied; I took her to the doctor, who told me that stomachaches were the commonest of childhood complaints, and that he could find nothing wrong with her. Eventually she stopped mentioning them.

But those hours and days and weeks of worry can't be so easily dispelled, even by a happy diagnosis from a pediatrician. At night I stand in their rooms and watch them sleep, their covers thrown off, arms and legs splayed across their sheets and blankets. Sometimes I raise my hand and make a sign of the cross in the air, a layman's blessing—first Katie, in the top bunk, then Madeleine below. Mostly I just stand and watch, knowing, too, that the days and years in which I have this privilege of watching my children sleep in perfect health may be numbered.

What disturbs my vision, especially after my time in the hospital, is imagining the children living through a similar ordeal, for any reason, or having to spend weeks or months laid up in bed. What a change from their lives of running and dancing and laughing it would be! How could they survive it? How could I survive it?

It was not until later in the year, during the driving vacation we took to visit our old home cities in the Midwest, that a kind of solution to both sides of this problem began to present itself to me. A solution of sorts—nothing, I understand, will ever remove my fears for my children, or, as they get older, their fears for me.

But I learned something, on that trip, that might help.

OVER THE COURSE of that trip we spent, in transit between Massachusetts and Cleveland, St. Louis, and Chicago, somewhere in the range of forty hours in the car. We did everything we could to make those hours more palatable for the girls. We bought them small toys to play with in the car; we carted a case of their dolls along; we packed their favorite CDs; we checked out from the library some children's books on tape; and we brought a shopping bag full of videos for the TV/VCR that came installed with our minivan. We tried always to make sure we were on the road during the hours after lunch, when body metabolism slows and even Katie is likely to take a nap if she's immobilized in her car seat.

But even with these precautions, it was impossible to banish all dead time from the car: those moments when the videos are giving them motion sickness, no one could stand another second of the soundtrack from *The Little Mermaid*, their dolls are scattered on the floor around them, and naptime is over.

So in those moments we did the only thing we could do: we stared out the windows. And, especially as we drove through the mountainous and tree-lined highways of Massachusetts and upstate New York, a memory of a childhood activity began to emerge from the fog of memories I have of my youth.

For many years the family vacations we took when I was a child were brief trips to a small lakeside cabin within a couple of hours from our home, and so did not involve excessive amounts of driving. But one year we drove from Cleveland to Florida over the course of three days, and for another few years we went to an island off the coast of South Carolina. We did not have the luxury of VCRs or even tape decks during those drives, and a propensity for motion sickness in my family prevented almost all of us from reading. So we fought with one another, and played travel games, and slept.

But as I drove with my own children through the window-staring hours, I gradually remembered how I had occupied those dead times when I was young, in an activity that fell somewhere between a game and a daydream.

I see very clearly now that this activity was the mental calisthenics of a budding writer. As we would drive through any particular landscape, I would picture myself suddenly set down in the midst of it, and imagine what might happen to me. Driving between the dynamite-blasted walls of a mountain, I would watch myself meticulously climbing the rocks, away from the speeding cars to the safety of the woods. In the fields of Midwestern farms, I would see myself threading my way through a herd of cows, in search of a farmer who could help me find my way back to my family. In the cities I saw myself set down at a busy intersection, alone and lost among the tall buildings and crush of horn-blowing cars. Dropped into the midst of a forest in a valley, I would find a running stream of water and follow it to civilization.

The nature of my imaginative flights from the car eventually evolved from these hypothetical survival narratives to the more enjoyable pastime of simply envisioning myself as a resident of any particular landscape. Now I was a farmer's son, rising every morning at the crack of dawn to milk the cows and collect the eggs from the henhouse; now I was a hiker alone on the mountain, cooking my food over an open fire and sleeping under the stars; now I was a boy who lived in an apartment in a city, and saw nothing but concrete and steel everywhere I turned.

At one point in this most recent vacation, I realized that these memories were returning to me because, in fact, I have never given up this imaginative exercise. I still play these games in my mind on long car trips. Before we set out for such a trip I usually will identify some intellectual problem I need to think through, so that I can use the time in the car productively—do some advance planning for a syllabus, for example, or decide upon the right ending for a piece of writing I am finishing. Instead of thinking diligently about these problems, my mind inevitably wanders away, seeking out shelters in the landscapes around me.

As we drove back to Massachussetts from Cleveland, I introduced my daughters, especially Katie, to this speculative exercise. At the time, I did not do it for any conscious purpose other than to help us pass the time in the car. It was easy enough to play this game as we drove through the mountainous terrain of upstate New York and western Massachusetts, passing by one spectacular vista after another along the Massachusetts Turnpike: imagine yourself at the top of that mountain, imagine yourself at the bottom of that one, imagine yourself on a boat in that river, imagine yourself living in that lonely farmhouse on the hillside there.

As we imagined our way through those landscapes, a series of linked ideas began to emerge and crystallize from the reflections on fatherhood I had been entertaining since my hospitalization. I started to see a link between what had helped me pull Madeleine back into my life, what I was teaching Katie on those car trips, and what I could offer to my children to help them cope both with my own illness and with—God forbid—any future illnesses of their own.

As a writer, I have probably always been aware that the greatest gift I can offer to my children is the imagination, and a full appreciation of the satisfaction that comes from artistic creation of any sort. That realization only came fully to my consciousness, though, as the long shadow cast by my hospitalization began to recede.

Now I see clearly how I can best be a father to the children of a chronically diseased man, one whose genes may one day put them at risk for that same chronic disease. I cope with my illness through my writing, as I describe more fully in the next chapter, and through the process of creating artistic order from the senselessness of disease. Writing helps me both work through the disease and escape from the disease.

I want my children, whether the time ever comes that they

need those skills or not, to be equipped with the imaginative and creative powers to help them cope with whatever trauma they may face in their lives. Gluing acorns on a badly drawn construction-paper tree models those creative powers at the most basic level, as does cultivating the ability to cast one's imagination out of a confined and closed space into the landscapes you will never touch, and perhaps never see again.

Before my hospitalization, I guided my children through those activities on instinct, from the common desire that all parents have to lead our children along the happier paths that we have followed; I do so deliberately now, nurturing their creative and imaginative powers with projects, with shared efforts at writing stories and poems and songs, with oral rhyming games and other word play, and with, above all, a constant modeling of my own love for books and the works of the creative imagination in any form.

Of course I want my children to take a healthy interest in the outdoors, in exercising their bodies, and in sports and normal childhood games. But most of all I want them to have the creative and imaginative resources to thrive and enjoy their lives, whatever fates their bodies hand to them.

As THIS LESSON became clear to me in the spring and early summer, I was able to soothe my anxieties about the genetic inheritance I might pass along to my children, and to turn with a willing heart to the task of trying to conceive our third child.

But I want to save that story, and its outcome, for the final chapter.

8

CARRYING OUR SECRET PAINS

Learning to Tell My Story

[April–May 2001]

Around eight years ago my mother was diagnosed with cancer in her tongue and her lymph nodes, and went through a successful course of surgery and radiation therapy to remove the growths. Still, though, she occasionally gets small growths beneath her tongue that require surgical removal; those removals have ranged from small outpatient procedures to skin grafts requiring reconstructive surgery. Her doctors have told her that she may continue to see these small growths for the rest of her life, but that they are treatable and should never become life-threatening, as long as they are closely monitored.

Maddeningly—at least to me—she often does not tell her children about these growths, and sometimes even the minor outpatient surgeries to remove them, until after they happen. Then she glosses over them quickly, letting us know via e-mail that she has seen the doctor and that everything turned out well.

"Mom," I will say to her afterward, frustrated, "I ask you every week how you are doing, and you never said anything about this new problem during the entire month you were worrying about it. Don't you think I really want to know how you're doing?"

"I know," she will respond simply. "I'm sorry."

During one of those discussions, I managed to squeeze a little more out of her about why she does this.

"I know you don't feel this way, Jimmy," she said to me over the phone one evening. "I know you understand what it's like. But most people don't want to hear about it when you're sick, or when you're worried about being sick."

"I know," I said.

"So when people ask me how I'm doing, I just tell them I'm doing fine. And that's what they want to hear. They want to hear I'm doing fine. People don't want to listen to me describing the little bump I discovered under my tongue last week, and hear me complain that I'm not sleeping at night because I'm so worried about it."

"You're right, Mom," I said. "I've had the same experiences. Just remember that I'm the exception. I *do* want to hear about it."

"I'll try to remember," she said.

As I reflected upon this conversation later that afternoon, it took me just a moment or two of self-analysis to realize that I was often guilty of the precise sin for which I was chastising my mother.

MY SISTER GOT MARRIED in October of 2000—around the time described in chapter four—the last sibling of the five of us to do so. We flew to Cleveland for the wedding, and at the reception

I had a chance to speak with members of my extended family whom I had not seen for many years.

One of those was my mother's brother, Uncle Mike, whose wife had recently died of cancer. I stopped to talk with him on my way to the bar for a drink, and he asked about my health. At that time I was taking quite a bit of medication, unsuccessfully trying to taper off prednisone and dealing with moderate disease activity, and I told him so. My mother had shared with him the details of my illness, so I probably offered him more detail than I would have to most friends or acquaintances who ask me about my health.

After hearing my health report, he made a sympathetic comment about the hassle of taking multiple daily medications. I responded with some version of the comment with which I almost always conclude narratives of my health and my medications:

"It was hard at first, but after a while you get used to it. It's not so bad anymore."

He smiled at me, and nodded.

"I'm sure that's what you tell people, Jim, but I know that's not really true."

I was momentarily taken aback at his response, but then recollected that he had spent the last year or two caring for his dying wife.

"You're right," I said. "But that's what I tell people."

I HAD BEEN TELLING PEOPLE that for five years, for several reasons.

Like most young people—even those of us as "young" as thirty-three—I had youth's fear and revulsion of infirmity and disease. Prior to my diagnosis, the malfunctioning and decay of the human body in any form repulsed me, no doubt because it reminded me of the fact that I, too, had a physical body that would one day suffer this fate.

I knew that other people shared these sentiments. I had seen them in the way that children, and even college students, react to physical decay and disease. Students in my writing classes will often write essays about their first experiences with death, as they have watched their grandparents die. Those essays frequently describe the mixed feelings students have at reconciling their love for their grandparents with their revulsion at dealing with a decayed and diseased human body.

I have a nightmarish series of memories of this sort: a collection of mental slides of the death of my grandfather, including— hitting far too close to home—a scene in which he has shat himself, and is calling both plaintively and angrily to my grandmother to come and change him; another of him, frail and emaciated, in a nursing home bed, unable to remember or recognize me—me, who had for many years privately bestowed upon him that important childhood honor of favorite grandparent.

So my primary fear was that any revelations I made about my condition would cause others to see me, first and foremost, as a diseased body. I knew what could accompany that perception: the unpleasant reflections on the parts of our physical selves that we do our best to ignore, and the fear of our own mortality. I had felt those same emotions myself, in the face of others' pains and illnesses.

But I was also afraid that even those people who might not find the diseased body repulsive might still brand me with that label, and that prospect was equally unpleasant to me. I was afraid that, for most people, I would be lodged in their minds as "the guy with Crohn's disease."

That label captured the one part of me that I wanted to dissociate myself from. Label me the Professor, the Father-with-Two-Children, the Writer, the Brother and Son, label me Quick-Tempered, Lazy-about-Housework, Struggles-with-Alcohol, Occasionally Self-Centered—label me as anything but Man-with-Crohn's-Disease. No single label could encapsulate what seemed most essential to my self, but the disease label seemed to me especially distant from the parts of myself in which I could take some pride and satisfaction.

So, for five years I had been doing my best to conceal the actual nature and extent of my illness from both friends and colleagues at school. Of course my family knew, and some of our closest friends, but I tried to minimize the number of people who were fully aware of my condition. When I was ill I relied on the stock phrase "I wasn't feeling well"; if I needed to explain in more detail a prolonged bout of sickness, I simply said that I had "stomach problems."

Even then, I knew I was doing precisely what so angered me when I read about others coping with the disease—papering over my illness and its symptoms with easy euphemisms. But that didn't stop me from turning around and using those euphemisms when I was confronted with an acquaintance curious about my health.

I maintained this strategy of denial and evasion even as late as my stay in the hospital, when—you would think—I would no longer be able to hide the nature of my condition. But remember that e-mail I sent to my colleagues from my hospital bed, asking them to help me with my classes? Here is the paragraph in which I described what had put me in the hospital:

I am in the hospital at the moment, and will be here at least until Wednesday. I expect to be out on that day, and back in the classroom either on Friday or Monday. FYI, I came down with

an awful stomach virus last Monday, which put me in the hospital on Monday night and Wednesday night—only to come again
on the following day each time. Mistake. I am now in here for a
little bit of a duration—the stomach virus triggered some other
problems, and I am getting IV fluids and medicine for a few days
until it has all settled down.

"Some other problems": five years of illness, five years of multiple
medications a day, five years of anxiety and concern about my
health, five different gastroenterologists, three colonoscopies, one
week in the hospital, all rolled into that innocuous little phrase.

"Some other problems." No phrase could capture more perfectly the extent to which I would seek out meaningless phrases to
describe my illness to others. Anything that avoided reference to
the chronic nature of the problem would do; anything that avoided
reference to the specific nature of the disease was absolutely necessary. Stomach viruses were acceptable; inflamed colons were not.

And this leads to the final reason I did my best to conceal the
disease from others—the fact that the primary symptom of this
disease, at least in my case, is one that we don't discuss in contemporary American society.

Proof of the silence our culture steadfastly maintains about
diarrhea is most apparent in television commercials for antidiarrheal medications. Most of the time, those commercials won't even
mention the word diarrhea until the final few seconds, when a picture of the medication comes onto the screen—if they even mention it at all. They tend to play out like this:

> SCENE: Good-looking man and wife are dressing for a party. The
> man suddenly sits down on the bed, bow tie hanging over his
> tuxedo shirt, and says to his wife:
> MAN: I don't think I can make it tonight, honey.

WOMAN (making a face): Is it . . . ?

MAN (nodding ruefully): Yes.

An announcer breaks in to explain authoritatively how the medication coats the lining of the stomach and intestines with soothing medicine, providing relief—from what?—for up to twelve hours. Cut back to . . .

SCENE: Man and woman are standing together at a formal party, laughing happily. FADE OUT . . .

The woman's pained expression, her inability to complete the question—to use the actual word—reflects one of our society's great taboos: we do not, in public, discuss our shit.

I have found the best explanation for this social taboo in the work of a now-deceased philosopher and psychologist named Earnest Becker, whose Pulitzer Prize–winning book, *The Denial of Death*, I first encountered as an undergraduate—at precisely the time when I was experiencing my first regular and sustained bouts of diarrhea. Those bouts were nothing like what I experienced in the weeks preceding my diagnosis in 1996, but I suspect they were the first manifestations of the disease. At the time, I attributed the diarrhea to dining hall food and too much beer. But, whatever the cause, the diarrhea I was experiencing at that time no doubt highlighted for me the lessons Becker has to teach about the meaning of shit in the human condition.

Becker argues that human excrement reminds us of two features of the human condition that we all would like to ignore: the limitations of our human aspirations to intellectual and spiritual achievement, and the inevitability of our physical death and decay.

Describing the paradox of humanity succinctly and eloquently, Becker calls the human animal "the god that shits." We are godlike in what we have achieved in spiritual and intellectual matters: the finest works of art and literature, the amazing advancements in science and technology, and the moral heroics of our earthly saints. But however lofty our intellectual and spiritual ambitions may be, however incredible our achievements, we all must acknowledge our identity and limitations as human bodies when we are on the toilet. When Michelangelo descended from the ceiling of the Sistine Chapel to move his bowels, he shared the fate, if not the actual toilet, of the meanest of Italian peasants—not to mention our own fates as well.

Excretion reveals to us too that our free will, as human animals, is limited by our bodies. Although we have basic bodily needs in many areas—such as the needs for food, drink, oxygen, and warmth—those are all needs we can in fact choose to ignore. Ignoring such physical necessities might lead to our own self-destruction, but we are perfectly capable of making that choice. I may refuse food and drink, and I may choose to end my own life by depriving myself of oxygen.

Not so with excretion. Excretion makes its demands upon the body, and requires that we subject ourselves to its whims, at least momentarily. Although we may be able to postpone the body's demand to excrete, we must succumb to it eventually. It is for this reason that Becker places excretion at the focal point of the conflict between our physical bodies and our spiritual and intellectual values:

> Nature's values are bodily values, human values are mental values, and though they take the loftiest flights they are built upon excrement, impossible without it, always brought back to it . . . The anus and its incomprehensible, repulsive product represents not only physical determinism and boundness, but the fate as well of all that is physical: decay and death. (31)

When we excrete, we acknowledge the submission of ourselves to the natural world's cycle of birth, decay, and death. This natural cycle exists and perpetuates itself without our formal consent—it pre-existed us, it controls a significant portion of our daily lives, and it will outlast us. Shitting is the closest and most frequent contact most of us have with the fundamental paradox of being human, caught between the world of physical necessity—and its attendant features of decay and death—and the world of spirituality and intellect.

I am not suggesting, of course, that the advertising executives who manage the antidiarrheal medication accounts discuss these ideas at their television commercial brainstorming sessions. But that is precisely the point: These are revelations about the human condition that we don't want to hear. They are buried deep in our minds, deep enough that we are capable of forgetting them through the course of our daily lives. We do our best to ignore anything that reminds us of them.

All this philosophical theorizing leads to two basic points: Those of us with chronic illness of any sort are often reluctant to tell our stories, for fear of how they will impact the perceptions of those around us; those of us with inflammatory bowel diseases bear the extra burden of knowing that offering even the most simple, truthful explanation of our illnesses and their symptoms inspires discomfort and unease in our listeners.

So we learn, quickly enough, to keep our stories to ourselves. It is a lesson that sinks in, so much so that even when I am confident I will find in someone a sympathetic ear, I usually remain silent.

When we first moved to Worcester in August, our neighborhood had a block party, attended by at least a hundred of our new neighbors. This took place in late August or early September, during the time that I was just beginning to receive medicinal help for the disease, so I was still experiencing disease activity.

The party was one street over from ours, which meant that I had to walk two blocks back to our house when I needed a bathroom.

At one point during the party, while Anne and I were talking to several of our new neighbors, I suddenly felt some pressure on my bowels.

"I need to grab something at the house—I'll be right back," I said to the group, and excused myself.

Later, after I had returned, one of the neighbors with whom I had been speaking when this happened approached me.

"My sister has Crohn's disease," she said. "So how are you doing?"

I was taken aback. How did she know? I realized after a moment's thought that Anne must have said something about it to the group after I had excused myself.

Given this neighbor's obvious knowledge of the disease, and the likelihood that she would have some understanding of, and empathy for, my situation, I could have been honest with her easily. I wanted to be honest with her. But it was as if some barrier had formed in my mouth, a filter through which the truth could not escape. Instead, I pushed the "Play" button on the tape recorder:

"I'm doing fine," I said. "I have a pretty mild case of the disease."

Later, back at home, I chided Anne for what she had done.

"I would prefer to keep the disease to myself," I told her.

"Why? I didn't think it was a big deal."

"It is to me. I just would prefer to keep it to ourselves. I don't really like having to tell everyone all about it and explain everything. It's embarrassing. Just let me tell people if I decide I want to tell anyone."

"Okay," she said, with a shrug.

OF COURSE, while I would not allow myself—or my wife—to talk about my disease with anyone, I was desperate to do precisely that.

Like anyone with a chronic illness, at times I wanted to feel the sympathy of others. I wanted other people to understand what I was experiencing, to recognize the extent of my suffering, to offer me comfort and support. At times I wanted to share my sorrows with others so that I could learn if anyone else was undergoing similar experiences.

No matter how desperately I wanted these things, though, I could not budge that filter I had installed in my mind and my mouth, the one that either hid the disease from others or sugar-coated the realities of it.

I could not budge it myself; my stay in the hospital, fortunately, did it for me.

MY CONVERSATIONS with others who had Crohn's disease had been extremely limited up to that point. After I was diagnosed, my mother passed along the phone number of a family friend who had, upon her diagnosis many years ago, had a complete colectomy. I spoke with her once on the telephone, to get some advice about gaining weight after one of my flares. My wife's aunt and uncle lived next door to a woman with Crohn's; I had a very brief conversation with her once in the driveway of her home.

Beyond these experiences, all of my contact with fellow sufferers had been through print—books, magazines, the Internet.

While I was in the hospital, I was visited every eight hours by a technician who would take my blood pressure, check my temperature, and record the information on a chart. It was usually a different technician at each shift.

One afternoon, a day or two before I was released, a short, thin woman with long and dark curly hair knocked and wheeled in the familiar cart. This was her first visit to me.

"Are you the one with Crohn's disease?" she asked me. She had a thick Massachusetts accent.

I nodded.

"I have it, too."

"Really? Where do you have it?"

"Small intestine."

The symptoms of the disease can vary widely, depending upon which part of the digestive tract it strikes. Only around 20 percent of Crohn's patients have it exclusively in the colon, as I do; most people have it in the final third of their small intestines. For those people—unlike myself—abdominal pain is often the worst symptom of the disease.

This was the case with the technician, who took pain medication, and had had two surgeries to remove pieces of her small intestine that had been causing her significant problems.

I know this because she told me her story in the hospital room that day, and—for the first time—I told her mine. It must have been a combination of circumstances that loosened my lips: the fact that I knew she would understand my experiences; the fact that we were in a medical setting, even though she was not my doctor or nurse; and the fact that I had spent the last five days in a hospital bed, weakened physically and mentally, and anxious about my future.

By the time she left I felt, at least mentally, markedly better than I had before her arrival. I understood that this lift in my spirits resulted from our conversation, and from the opportunity I had to speak openly with another about my disease. I had been given a glimpse into her life with disease, and I had given her a glimpse into mine. Those glimpses helped me to recognize the value of our exchange, both the listening and the telling.

In the listening I heard a story of suffering comparable to my own. I heard about experiences against which I could measure my own, both favorably and unfavorably. Seeing my experiences in the light of another's was illuminating; it helped me see how normal and routine, for other Crohn's sufferers, was much of what seemed to me, in my isolation, so exceptional and unbearable.

In the telling I was able to shape my experiences, to put them in the form of a narrative that made sense to me. It is through stories that we make sense of our lives, and the experience of disease is no different. We are hard-wired, as human beings, to create order from the chaos of our daily experience through the narratives we tell each other about the courses of our lives. Those narratives place the events of our lives in meaningful sequences.

Telling my story in the hospital helped me begin to do that with my disease. Both in the telling itself, and in the reflecting upon that telling afterward, I began to see for the first time how I had been following a pattern of delaying treatment until it was too late, how my worst experiences with disease seemed to come after I had stalled and hesitated my way into serious flares. I began to wonder what other patterns might emerge from telling a more detailed version of my story, what other lessons I might learn myself and perhaps share with others. Lying in that hospital bed, it became clear to me for the first time that I had to construct this very narrative, the one you hold in your hands, to tell my story both for my own sake—to give you a glimpse into my darkness—but for the sake of others as well, to help them understand how that telling brings both comfort and meaning to an otherwise chaotic and meaningless experience.

And so in the weeks following my hospital stay, in addition to the slow work I began to do on this story, I became more open about my condition with those around me, beginning at school.

Early one morning I mustered my courage and sat down with my department chair in her office to explain to her exactly what was wrong with me. As other colleagues stopped me in the hallway to check on my health, once I had returned to work, I let myself name my condition to them, and offered simple explanations of the disease's most basic features.

It was this newfound openness, this willingness to tell my own story, that led me to confront a version of my pre-hospital self, a meeting that convinced me even more thoroughly how important it was for me to tell my own story.

IN THE LATE SPRING, another professor in my department approached me to discuss a student who had been having some trouble in his class. This student had been missing classes recently, and the quality of his work had suffered a marked decline from the beginning of the semester to that point, which was just a week or two away from finals.

Once he had called the student into his office to discuss his work in the course, my colleague had discovered that the student had been ill for much of the semester, and had been shuttling back and forth between doctors who initially were baffled by his symptoms. Eventually, though, the possibility of Crohn's disease had been broached to him, and by the time my colleague approached me the tests that would help confirm that diagnosis had already been performed.

In his conversation with the student, my colleague could tell that he was in a state of complete emotional turbulence, and was terrified at the possibility of this diagnosis. My colleague had approached me to see whether I might meet with the student to discuss his concerns, answer any questions he might have about the disease, and provide a positive example of someone who was living with it.

Of course I agreed, and a few days later my colleague ushered a very large—both tall and stout—young man into my office. At first I thought there must be some mistake, because Crohn's disease almost always produces weight loss. I learned later that, in some rare cases, the disease—depending upon the precise location of the inflammation within the intestinal tract—can have the opposite effect, and can produce weight gain.

I invited him to sit down, and asked him to tell me his story.

"Well, I've been sick," he said. "And they think it's Crohn's disease."

"What sort of symptoms have you been having?"

"Stomach pain. Really terrible stomach pains, especially after I eat."

"Anything else?"

"Mostly the stomach pains."

"No diarrhea?"

"Oh, yeah—that too. After I eat."

"Anything else?"

"Mostly those things."

And so it went, for ten or fifteen minutes—me prompting him to tell me his story, and he refusing to offer me anything more than the most basic information about his condition, giving me even that somewhat reluctantly.

I found it maddeningly frustrating. Flush with my new awareness of the importance of sharing my story with others, I wanted him to tell me *his* story—to describe for me what his life had been like up to that point, to narrate the onset of his symptoms, and to describe his current condition in as much detail as possible. I wanted all of this information because it would have helped me to compare our experiences, and to decide what sorts of information, advice, and perspective I might most usefully give to him. But I also wanted to do him the service of offering him a sympathetic ear, a sounding board against which he could begin to organize the undoubtedly chaotic events of the past few months into some kind of order.

But his filters were already too firmly stuck in place. Eventually I gave up, and simply began to tell him everything about the disease that I wished I had been told after my own diagnosis. At the end of it, he said I had answered all of the questions he had, and he thanked me for my time. I told him to please get in touch with me again if he had any additional concerns, and to stop by my office at any time.

I haven't seen him since.

Of course I understood, even then, that he was behaving in a perfectly normal manner—behaving as I would have behaved in his position just a few months earlier. He understood that you do not discuss your malfunctioning body with strangers. He understood that you do not just open up and tell your disease story to anyone who asks how you are doing. And an eighteen-year-old college student, above all, does not sit in the office of a professor and talk— however persistently the professor questions him—about the frequency or consistency of his bowel movements.

My encounter with this student was perhaps the first instance in which I sought out the disease story of a stranger. Since then, I have undertaken this process more actively, and now seek out such stories wherever I can find them. I do so partly in order to provide me with new perspectives on living and coping with my own chronic illness, and partly to help others experience the same sense of satisfaction and release that has accompanied the telling of my own story.

No doubt I could have come to this lesson far more easily and quickly by taking advantage of a local Crohn's disease support group. One exists at my local hospital. I would certainly recommend to others, especially to those who may not be as inclined as I am to put their narratives on paper, to take advantage of these opportunities to tell their stories and hear the stories of others.

Support groups are simply not for me, and I suspect I am not alone in this respect. I am better at one-on-one conversations, or in classroom situations in which I can direct and control the conversation. I have a harder time finding my voice in the more unstructured and egalitarian setting of the support group.

So I will continue to put my own story down on paper, if for no other reason than to help me continue to make sense of it. I will seek out the stories of others in the best ways I know how to elicit them.

RECENTLY I WAS ATTENDING an academic conference with a friend whom I hadn't seen since I was diagnosed. I told him my story; when I was done, he told me his. He had a degenerative condition in his hands that prevented him from typing and writing, and he was slowly losing the strength of his grip. Though I had known him for several years, I had never known about this condition, and I commented upon that.

"We all carry around our secret pains," he said to me afterward, sighing.

Chronic illness has taught me to see, to understand, and to respect the secret pains of others. It has taught me, as well, to make my own pains a little less secret.

UNBURDENING MYSELF of my secret pains, though, remains difficult, however beneficial I know the telling of my story can be.

Part of that difficulty stems from the lingering reluctance I have to be labeled, and to air in public what at least some of my listeners no doubt would prefer that I keep private. But after five years with the disease, part of that difficulty now comes from the accumulation of emotion that has built up around the story.

Telling my story means, in a very small way, reliving experiences that have been extremely difficult for me, both physically and emotionally. Telling my story means rehashing events that I often wish I could forget.

The writing, editing, and even final proofreading of almost every chapter in this book has found me, at one point or another, sitting on the couch next to the computer in my basement, crying shamelessly—lamenting the past, fearing the future—and trying to forget everything I have been describing in this book. The pages of this manuscript have been stained, metaphorically and sometimes quite literally, with my tears.

What those tears are calling for is simple enough: They want me to put this year behind me, they want me to think only of the future, they want me to dream of a future in which this past will never have existed, will be like a nightmare from which I have now awakened. They want me to forget my story, and to begin my life anew.

But I cannot forget, however healthy I am. Cannot and must not.

I am learning to tell this story.

9

TIME PASSES

Learning to Be Healthy

[Summer 2001]

Learning to be healthy, like all of the learning experiences I have described in this book, has not been the sort of lesson I could achieve in a moment of revelation and then file away. Learning to be healthy has been an ongoing challenge for me, one that has stretched from the days following my hospital stay to the moment I am typing these words. Learning to be healthy has not gotten one bit easier, and I don't expect it to get any easier.

I can demonstrate this most clearly by describing how I learned to curb my daily drinking.

I HAVE STRUGGLED with alcohol since my very first taste of it— two or three bottles from a twelve-pack of Michelob Light, choked down in the backseat of a station wagon on the way to a U2 concert with Tony and some friends of ours during my sophomore year of high school. It was a night of firsts for the Lang brothers: I drank my first beer, and Tony smoked his first joint.

Tony's first contact with marijuana didn't make much of an impression on him and never developed into a habit. In this, as in many other ways in which Tony has preceded me in eventually shared experiences, I wish I had followed his wise example.

Shortly after that first taste of beer, I began drinking at every opportunity possible. Such opportunities were relatively infrequent for an academically motivated suburban kid who came from a large family with a mother who stayed at home and kept strict tabs on our comings and goings. But by my junior year of high school I was out most weekend nights, pouring as much beer down my gullet as I could between the time I left home and my curfew hour. I made friends with peers who had similar habits, and we encouraged each other in our shared vice.

In college, with parental supervision lifted, I drank a little bit more each semester, and carried my habits home with me on breaks. During the summer between my sophomore and junior years of college, this came to a head one Sunday morning after a particularly bad Saturday night.

I had come in so late that my parents had not bothered to wake me for church—an absolutely unprecedented event in our household. When they returned, my father summoned me out onto our back porch, and we sat on the steps, both of us looking out into the backyard. The sun was shining on a warm July day, and I could still feel the alcohol in my system, giving everything around me a sense of unreality. My father was not angry, as I expected him to be. He seemed confused, like a man confronted with a problem he simply did not know how to resolve.

"Jim," he said to me slowly. "Your mother and I would like you to give up drinking for a week."

"Okay," I said, grateful to be let off so easily.

And that was all they asked.

And that was all I did. I gave up drinking for one week. I told my friends that I wasn't going out that week, and I stayed in every night and read. That didn't satisfy my mother, who insisted that I needed to learn how to go out with my friends and still not drink. I knew that, however, was impossible. But I had still fulfilled their request to the letter. When the week was completed, I gradually resumed my old habits.

I suspect I could easily have lost control in a more serious way if I had not met Anne a month into my junior year of college. In the weeks before I met her, I remember going out with some friends for lunch on a Sunday after a long weekend of drinking, and ordering one of the restaurant's extra-large mugs of beer. The next thing I knew I was asleep on the couch in my room. I awoke to find a note, scrawled on a piece of cardboard and pinned to my chest, from the two girls I had been with, describing how they had to drag me home and pour me onto my dorm-room couch after I had begun nodding off at lunch. I remember going to the late-night Catholic mass in my dorm's chapel that evening, sitting by myself and wondering whether I had traveled so far down the road to alcoholism that I would need professional help getting back.

A few weeks later I met Anne, and my relationship with her became serious very quickly. Both she, and the importance of that relationship to me, helped temper the worst excesses of my drinking. I renewed my academic work with vigor, and studied my way back onto the dean's list that semester, after the mediocre grades of my sophomore year.

But if I kept better control of myself for the remainder of my college years, and in the early years of our marriage that followed, it didn't mean I drank any less. I simply drank more regularly. So regularly, in fact, that by the time I graduated from college and had moved on to graduate school, I had settled into the very regular and steady habit of drinking three beers every night before I went to bed.

That habit lasted from my senior year of college until my stay in the hospital, with perhaps—over the course of those ten years— two or three dozen days on which I did not have at least one alcoholic beverage to drink.

Of course I had no good reason to drink. My parents and siblings all loved me, I had material comforts, and I had lived a childhood of security and support that most people would envy. Neither of my parents drank excessively; my mother was, and remains, a near-teetotaller, while my father would have a few drinks at parties, or perhaps a drink when he came home from work. I was always an A student, with a strong love of literature and writing, and my academic success was praised and rewarded both at home and in school.

Thus any psychological angst I could claim to have driven me to drink would have been completely self-induced.

That doesn't make my struggles with alcohol, which continue to this day, any less real. Looking back, I am convinced that I settled on the habit of drinking three beers every night before bed as a means of keeping my drinking in check. As long as I had a strict routine, one that limited my daily intake to an amount that did not cause me either hangovers or serious health problems, I could continue to drink without losing control.

But the best evidence that this strategy does not preclude my being, at the very least, a problem drinker was that except for the absolute nadirs of my flare-ups, I continued to drink without interruption throughout all of my illnesses.

If I had no good reason to drink before the spring of 1996, I certainly felt justified in my drinking after that. I had a chronic illness, after all—I was suffering physically and mentally. Drinking helped me cope, drinking helped me forget, drinking helped me feel like I was twenty years old again, the owner of a healthy body that could withstand any sort of gastrointestinal pounding I pushed it to endure.

Never mind the fact that drinking three or more beers every day will loosen anyone's bowels a bit, especially mine, and never mind that the alcohol probably interfered with the effects of some of the medications I took. My gastroenterologists had assured me that nothing that passed between my lips could affect the course of the disease, and that assurance provided me with the excuse I needed to continue drinking.

If anything, the development of the disease entrenched me all the more firmly in my habit of capping off the day with those nightly beers. The arrival of my children, which had coincided with the onset of my disease, had pretty much reduced or eliminated those occasions on which I could stay up late into the evening drinking at parties or in bars, unconcerned about the effects such behavior would have on me when I woke the following afternoon. The severely limited opportunities I had for binge drinking intensified my commitment to my milder habit of nightly drinking.

I tend to latch onto routines in my private life and then stick to them tenaciously. My nightly drinking thus became wrapped up into the routine of relaxation and unwinding I had developed to help me finish the day.

During the semester I am often at work on reading or writing or preparing for class until eleven o'clock in the evening. At that point, I close my book or shut down the computer and crack my first beer. I flop onto the couch, turn the television to whatever sitcom happens to be in the syndication schedule at that hour, and open the newspaper. I never have much energy for the news section; this is the point in the day when I am trying to relax my brain, and I spend much more time poring over sports scores and reading the comics than I do analyzing world politics.

The combination of the mindless banter of the television, the mindless content of the paper, and the mind-numbing effects of the alcohol gradually allow me to decompress, washing away the concerns of the day. It takes an hour to drink all three of the beers I have set aside for the evening, and by the time I am finished I am exhausted and fully ready for sleep.

I DRANK THE LAST OF my nightly beers on Sunday, February 11, 2001. I was sick at that time, of course, in the mode of moderate disease activity that had been plaguing me since December. But the next day, Monday, at around dinnertime, after I had eaten a light dinner and had drunk a glass of Gatorade to keep myself hydrated, I began experiencing the severe vomiting and diarrhea that would eventually land me in the hospital.

I had no choice but to stop drinking at that point. I couldn't keep any food in my stomach for several days, and by the time I was able to keep anything down I was in the hospital. When I got out of the hospital I was taking so many medications, and so much prednisone, that I was afraid to drink.

But even at that point, I had every intention of returning to my old habits. I left the hospital taking eighty milligrams of prednisone a day, with instructions to reduce to forty milligrams (a dose I was more accustomed to) within the next four weeks. I vowed to avoid alcohol until I had reduced to that dose; I held out the promise to myself that I would allow myself to drink again at that point.

Those four weeks were the longest I had ever gone without a

drink in my adult life. It was not as difficult for me as I would have expected, because I was so exhausted from the illness that I generally fell asleep as soon as I lay down on the couch after we had put the children to bed, and I crawled into bed before 10:00 PM on most nights. I did not need my evening routine to help me decompress and prepare for sleep; the disease was doing that for me.

But after those initial four weeks, I still had not reduced to forty milligrams of prednisone per day. That didn't happen for another two weeks. I planned my reduction in those final two weeks so that I would get to forty milligrams on a Friday; I would celebrate the weekend and my return to a familiar level of medication at the same time.

The day of reduction finally arrived, and my health was steadily improving. That evening I held off until my usual hour, 11:00 PM, and sat down on the couch with the first beer I had touched in six weeks. Six weeks. Watching the tiny bubbles foaming to the surface of the glass, I could hardly believe that it had been that long. I had not been dry for that long since my sophomore year of high school—fifteen years ago.

I reflected for a few minutes before I took that first sip. For the past few weeks, even as I recovered my strength and energy, I had been sleeping at night better than I used to. My three nightly drinks always knocked me out for the first few hours of the evening, but I usually woke up between 4:00 and 5:00 AM, dehydrated, and then drifted in and out of sleep until it was time to get up. Without the alcohol, I found myself sleeping until something besides my own body—an alarm clock, the girls, or a cat—woke me.

For most of my adult life, I had yearned for a nap every day. Most people want to nod off when the body's metabolism slows down in the early afternoon; I was ready to head back to bed at any point during the day. Since I had not been drinking, I found that I had more energy during the day. I no longer begged Anne to let me catch a quick nap on Saturday and Sunday afternoons, and I was no longer tempted to sleep for thirty minutes between classes in the easy chair in my office. I had energy during the day, and was tired enough in the evening that I fell asleep without much trouble.

I found I actually began to enjoy the mornings when I had not drunk alcohol the evening before. I did not snap at the children, I had an appetite for breakfast, and I had better control of my bowels. The morning had been transformed from a time period through which I tended to sleepwalk to one of the parts of the day that I actually enjoyed.

These changes had clearly improved the quality of my life; I could see that easily. Did I really want to take that sip?

Of course I wanted it, and I took it. It tasted funny to me, but I choked it down, and drank the two more I had brought out after it. By the time I was finishing the third one, it tasted a whole lot better.

I couldn't hold off that Friday evening; I had built that moment up—my triumphant return to alcohol—for too long in my mind. But that evening I fell into my customary sleep pattern: I awoke at 4:30 AM, thirsty, and got a glass of water. I tossed and turned in bed for two hours, and drifted off to sleep again sometime between 6:30 and 7:00 AM—just about an hour before I had to get up and get Katie off to her swimming lessons. That day, for the first time in a while, I sneaked upstairs for a nap while Anne took the girls out shopping. I was tired.

I found myself unable to resist the lure again on Saturday night; the association of alcohol and weekend nights was simply too strong for me to alter. But I did manage to scale back to just one beer on Sunday evening. On Monday, Tuesday, and Wednesday I had none.

For the next few weeks, in April and early May, I maintained this pattern. I kept myself dry Sunday through Wednesday; I allowed myself a beer or two on Thursdays, and I reverted to my old habits on Friday and Saturday.

In the meantime, I was slowly dropping the prednisone—from forty milligrams a day to thirty, to twenty, and then in slower increments to fifteen, ten, five. I had gradually eliminated Cipro from the medications I was taking. My bowel health was taking on a new character, and it was evident now that the Imuran had begun working. I would have three or four bowel movements in the morning, all within an hour of waking, and all diarrhea—but then I would be done for the day. I could actually spend the majority of my day living my life and not have to worry about being continually on the watch for restrooms. I no longer saw any blood in the toilet, and my strength and energy were now back to where they had been the previous summer.

In May I saw my gastroenterologist and described what I had been experiencing. He reduced the amount of Asacol I was taking every day from twelve pills to eight, and this cleared up my diarrhea within the space of a week.

The best part was that school was finishing, and I had the summer before me—the first summer I would have, since high school, in which I was not working at least part-time, and to which I could devote myself entirely to my two great joys: my family and my writing. I would also be able to relax my mind and release the stress that had been accumulating in my brain for the past nine months of my freshman year as an assistant professor, and for the past nine months of illness.

I could hardly allow myself to open my eyes to it, after the nine months I had lived through, but as school wrapped up in the third week of May, and spring was finishing its preparations for what

promised to be a glorious summer, I was beginning to believe that
a new era of remission and good health was on the horizon.

And that, of course, is precisely when the headaches and fevers
began.

I WAS CERTAIN, at first, that I had a cavity. I initially became
aware of a problem when I began to get sharp headaches, with the
pain localized in my upper jaw or behind my eye. They started off
slowly, but then worsened over the course of two weeks to the
point that I had to take aspirin at night to get to sleep.

At the same time, I developed a continuous, low-grade fever.
These fevers never reached the levels of the fevers I had experienced in the period before my diagnosis; at most, they would peak
at 102 degrees. Usually, they stayed in the range of 100–101. Like
all fevers, they were worse in the afternoon and early evening. I
became obsessed with monitoring my temperature, and took it
constantly. Typically I would be fine until at least lunchtime; by
2:00 PM the fever would be gradually moving into the 100-degree
range, and it reached its peak between 4:00 and 6:00 PM.

Was it possible that a cavity could cause a fever? I reasoned
myself into believing it was. I generally carried what I learned from
my disease about doctors and medicines into other areas of medical
care, and one day I had spent some time asking my dentist about
teeth and their care. He had explained the basics of his profession
to me eagerly, as if he had been waiting for someone to ask him
just these sorts of questions, and one of the points he had made
was that tooth decay was actually a bacterial infection.

Pain in my upper jaw, a fever to fight off an infection—massive
tooth decay, right? The problem was that I had no other symptoms
of a cavity: none of the teeth in the upper jaw were sensitive to the
touch, and hot and cold liquids did not increase the pain in any

way. The dentist I saw two weeks into this new problem pointed all this out to me, though I had known it myself, and suggested that my problem could involve the sinuses. He suggested that I consult my regular physician to try an antibiotic for a sinus infection.

That I did, and Dr. Honig seconded the diagnosis and prescribed an antibiotic. It didn't work. After ten days on that antibiotic, we tried a different one. It didn't work either. At this point nearly five weeks had passed, and I was still having the same regular fevers and head pain.

Fortunately, summer had arrived, and I was finished with school. Anne and Katie still had another six weeks of elementary school, and Madeleine was going to her sitter for six hours during the day so I could write. With the help of aspirin, I could write through most mornings. But I had little energy, and I was starting to get worried.

In the back of my mind loomed the diagnosis that I was becoming more and more concerned about, given that I was having unexplained head pain: a brain tumor of some sort. I did not discuss this fear with anyone, but as the days passed and the antibiotics failed to help, it seemed more and more likely to me.

Finally, late one evening I did an Internet search on brain tumors, and read as much as I could find. I was distressed to learn that headaches and fevers can, indeed, be common symptoms of brain tumors; I was somewhat relieved to discover that usually other symptoms accompany brain tumors—neurological symptoms like loss of coordination or vision problems. Still, I knew better than anyone how the body does not conform to what medical books—or Internet sites—say that it should be doing, and so the possibility remained in my mind.

Dr. Honig's eventual recommendation that I get a CAT scan of my sinuses did not help matters any. I wondered if he were using the language of investigating my sinuses in order to cover the fact that he was checking for head tumors of some sort.

My CAT scan appointment was at 7:00 one late June morning. I arrived on time and was immediately ushered into a room that contained a massive white ring, through which a bed on a track could pass. The nurse strapped me onto this bed, and then I was slowly jerked and pulled into position inside the ring. Somewhere inside that ring, something was spinning; I could hear the machine whirling around me, taking pictures of the inside of my skull in a way that I could not understand. The nurse told me not to move; I did my best to lie completely still. Of course I was worried that I might have to run to the bathroom at any moment, but fortunately this new problem—whatever it was—had not activated the disease in any way.

Suspended in the ring, eyes closed, the smell of medicine in my nostrils and the clicking and whirring of the scanner in my ears—all of it immediately brought me back to the hospital, and I thought of how easily I could be returned to that environment by an uncooperative body. I felt small and frail and out of control, a weak and sick body being processed through a machine, once again caught in the grip of the medical establishment in which I had little faith remaining.

It was over in fifteen minutes, and I was sent on my way, told that someone in the lab would read the results and convey them to my doctor. If they noticed something amiss, they would let him know immediately; if the results were routine, it might take longer for them to file the report.

So I found myself for a second time in a holding pattern, waiting nearly a week for test results that would define a condition that was interfering with my life in a significant way. I was not able to wait as long as I apparently was supposed to; I called the office a day or two early to see if the results had come in.

When Dr. Honig called me back later that same day he had news which, whatever he may have thought of it, seemed good to me: I had sinusitis in one sinus, and what looked like either inflammation or a polyp in the other. The word polyp initially shot up my cancer radar, but I was assured that sinus polyps were a common and benign condition. Later that week, while golfing with a neighbor who was a physician, I grilled him on my diagnosis and received confirmation of this.

If the sinuses continued not to respond to antibiotic treatment, eventually we would have to consider surgery. But Dr. Honig wanted to try one more kind of antibiotic before he sent me to a specialist.

And lo and behold, that last-chance antibiotic did the trick. Within a week of starting this final antibiotic the fevers had disappeared, and the headaches and facial pain were slowly receding. By the time I finished the antibiotic, and all of my symptoms had completely disappeared, six weeks of summer had passed me by.

Throughout those six weeks I had been forced to cut back on my drinking even further. I had noticed one day that my aspirin bottle contained a warning that people who regularly drink three or more alcoholic beverages a day should consult their physician before using any sort of pain reliever. It was a warning I would have ignored a year earlier; now, I decided it was best for me to just stop drinking so I could continue to take the aspirin that relieved the headaches and fever.

Once I had finished the antibiotic and felt myself cured of the sinus infection—although I was told that it could recur—I returned to my more limited drinking habits. I allowed myself beer on the weekends, but did my best to stay dry on weekdays. This was especially difficult during the summer, when I had no classes or office hours to get up for in the morning, but I forced myself to stick with my new regimen.

Put quite simply, what helped me in my resolve to cut back on my drinking was my rediscovery of the pleasures of living.

Roll Tape: Scenes in a Life Recovered

SCENE: Concord, Massachusetts, June. We have driven to this historic city outside of Boston and rented a canoe for a trip down the Concord River.

Anne and I situate ourselves at the ends of the canoe, with Katie and Madeleine, dwarfed by their oversized orange life preservers, on the benches between us. We push off from the dock and slowly paddle our way out into the river, toward our destination a mile or two down the river.

Though we started out with several other canoes, we round a bend and find ourselves alone, in the quiet of a short and isolated stretch of the river. Vegetation lines the banks on both sides of us, through which we can see houses in the distance. Suddenly, as if emerging from the river itself, a goose and six little goslings are paddling their way down the river beside us, perhaps a dozen feet from our canoe. We all notice them at once, and watch them in silence. The goslings paddle along quickly, rocking back and forth, behind their more smoothly gliding mother. Our canoe travels faster than they do; we slide past them quietly, and resume our paddling.

SCENE: Mid-morning, early July, on Chicago's Navy Pier, a promontory jutting into Lake Michigan from the heart of the city.

Anne, Katie, Madeleine, and I climb aboard the small red cars that will circle to the top of the 150-foot Ferris wheel—my sister, Peggy, who has accompanied us to the pier this morning, has decided to sit this one out. The wheel turns slowly, and we rise by inches to a place far above the pier, suspended and swaying lightly in the wind. I have a slight fear of heights, and this little gondola couldn't be more exposed. My heart beats quickly, and two or three small waves of panic come and go. I am gripping Katie fiercely by my side.

At the peak of the arc much of downtown Chicago is visible on my left; to the right, Lake Michigan stretches off into the horizon. The sky is clear, the day is warm, and the pier has begun to fill up with tourists like ourselves. They stroll casually around below us, some of them pointing up to the very car in which we sit. Out in the lake, I spot a yellow boat slipping over the waves, and I am hit with a desire to be on the water.

Down on the pier again, I buy us tickets for the *Sea Dog*—they are expensive, aimed at the captive market of tourists on the pier for the day, but I don't care—and we board the seventy-foot speedboat for a thirty-minute tour of the lakefront. Despite its large size, the boat reaches speeds of twenty-five knots, shooting spray into our faces and creating gusts of winds that feel like they will blow us right off the boat. This time it is Madeleine I am gripping tightly to my side. We rip across the surface of the lake, bouncing and sinking with the small waves, and I feel a powerful sense of freedom.

SCENE: Mid-July, a farm and vacation home in suburban St. Louis, owned by the family of Anne's sister's new boyfriend, Bruce, who both comes from money and has made a bunch of his own. We are in St. Louis on our three-week midwestern road trip, and have been invited out to the farm for a day of swimming, horseback riding, and relaxing.

After lunch and an early afternoon of swimming, Bruce rides from the farm up to the house on an ATV four-wheeler, one of those small, jeeplike vehicles that one steers and brakes like a bicycle, at the handlebars. He gives me directions to a pond we can see down in the valley below—their property stretches for acres in every direction—and I put Madeleine on the seat in front of me and take off, driving carefully over the path and out into the meadow that borders the pond.

Madeleine and I dismount and approach the edge of the pond, where we see tiny frogs hopping all around us. I catch one up in my hand and we admire it for just a moment before it hops away. We wander around at the edge of the pond, Madeleine chasing frogs and me watching Madeleine.

We return to the ATV and begin driving back across the meadow, but I stop at the sight of a greenish bump just off to one side of us. Sure enough, we have discovered a medium-sized box turtle. I pick him up and we watch him react, curling into his shell. Together we gently stroke the part of his back leg that remains exposed, feeling his tough, leathery skin. We admire the markings on his back.

Madeleine wants to bring him back to the house with us, but I say no.

"Let's leave him here," I say. "He would miss his friends and his home."

SCENE: Nantucket Island, thirty miles off Cape Cod in the Atlantic Ocean. Early August. Warm summer morning.

I load my bike and Katie's bike into our rented car, and Anne drives us from the vacation home we are renting on the island with another couple to a bike trail a half mile away. The road to the bike trail is narrow and usually filled with cars, and I don't trust Katie's fledgling bicycle-riding skills enough to let her negotiate the road alone.

The bike trail is wide and smooth, and crowded with bikers and walkers heading to and from the beach that sits about a mile from where we are donning our helmets and climbing onto our bikes. Katie starts off in the lead, pedaling hard to reach the speed she has decided is right for a bike ride with your dad. She weaves slightly back and forth when the trail is open, but when we approach other people or bikes she seems able to maintain her control, moving carefully to the edge to avoid collisions.

At the beach we put out bikes in the racks and I buy snow cones at the concession stand. We sit and watch people walking down the long sandy strip to the ocean.

Back on the bike trail again, I watch her slowly becoming more confident on her bike. She has just learned to ride by herself the week before this vacation, and she rides for the pure pleasure of it—for the joy of practicing and mastering a hard-won skill. I pedal slowly behind her, straining my ears to catch the constant stream of chatter that she keeps up throughout the ride. I don't hear most of it; I am content simply to watch and hear the sound of her voice.

"Okay," I keep shouting ahead. "Keep your eyes on the trail."

SCENE: An Audubon Society wildlife sanctuary, in Princeton, Massachusetts, just about twenty-five minutes from our home in Worcester. Mid-August. A thousand acres of hiking trails through meadows, woods, and ponds.

I searched this place out on the Internet, and brought Katie and Madeleine here one Friday afternoon. When we pull into the parking lot, we see sheep roaming around us. We stick a few dollars in the donation box, grab a trail map, and head off toward Beaver Pond. I am carrying Katie's school backpack—pink, with a picture of Snow White on the back—filled with snacks and sandwiches and the girls' wading boots.

We trek happily across a meadow and into the woods, up and down the sanctuary's rolling terrain until we arrive at the pond. The trail takes us to within a dozen feet of the beavers' huge lodge, packed in with mud and sticks and small trees. The girls clamor for their boots, and wade out into the shallow waters. They are ostensibly searching for frogs, but in reality they simply like the fact that they can put their feet into the water without getting into trouble.

We sit on the benches by the edge of the trail and eat our lunches, and then set off again. Their little legs are holding out well; they are exhilarated to find so much to see, to climb over and under, to run up and down. We walk a mile and a half to a tremendous boulder that, as the nearby plaque tells us, was pushed to this spot by a glacier some 15,000 years ago. We climb partway up it, and scream out "Hallos" to the woods around us, listening for the echoes. The girls want me to climb to the top of the boulder, which would require at least partially climbing a small tree. I am tempted, but then I remember I am thirty-two years old, and that I am here with my young children, and I decide against it.

I'll be back another day.

IN THE THREE MONTHS of that summer, I lived more intensely than I had in any other period of my life. I seized every possible new experience that crossed my path, devouring each one of them greedily.

I learned to be healthy that summer by giving up the daily

drinking that had held me for ten years and by beginning to exercise regularly and watch my diet more closely. I hope that I can retain all these habits.

But I think I can sum up what I learned from that summer in two simple lessons. When illness strikes, in any form, rest and make whatever sacrifices are necessary to return to health.

When health returns, live.

10

LEARNING HOPE, CAUTION, AND BALANCE

A Return to Daily Life

[August 2001]

Our destination is Good Harbor Beach in Gloucester, Massachusetts, approximately seventy-five miles, as the crow flies, from our home in Worcester. The journey, I have been assured by a neighbor who takes his children there regularly, will take us at least an hour and forty-five minutes. Packed into our minivan are Anne and me, Katie and Madeleine, and Mike, a fellow professor in the English department. Mike and I were hired at the same time by the college; we are office neighbors, fellow writers, and friends.

The end of August is approaching. The days have been long and beautiful, and promise to remain so for another few weeks at least. School holidays are about complete, and I have been slowly, sluggishly, turning my thoughts to school and to the upcoming year. I have been in the office a time or two already, preparing syllabi and doing some cleaning of my files. But I have been reluctant to really face the prospect of return. I am, first, mildly anxious that the return to school and work, with the stress that such a return will invariably create, will jeopardize my health again. But even more than that, I have enjoyed this summer with my wife and children as much as I can remember enjoying any time in my life, and I simply don't want it to end.

I banish thoughts of school from my head as we load up the car with blankets, beach toys, a cooler full of snacks and drinks, and extra clothes in preparation for our scheduled 9:00 AM departure.

I still don't enjoy mornings all that much, though they are no longer the trial for me that they had been just six months ago. I have settled into a happy routine: one or two bowel movements in the morning, shortly after awakening, and then no more for the rest of the day. Even as recently as March and April I would not have believed such a routine possible for me.

Minivan loaded, we pack into our seats and head out. We pick up Mike and are on the highway by 9:15, an amazingly timely start for us.

Mike, a bachelor, once made the mistake of cupping his hand and nipping at the girls' legs, pretending that he was a biting fish. He did not realize how quickly children grasp, and how long they hold onto, such familiar and easy games. Soon after we set off the girls begin giggling and protesting as loudly and unconvincingly as they can that they don't want any fish biting today.

Anne and I exchange looks and laugh, half at the children's simplistic duplicity, and half out of pity for Mike, who has sealed his fate with our children as the "Fishy" guy. He obliges them for several minutes, until Anne mercifully interrupts and offers the girls several choices of music on the car ride.

We sail along to the melodious strains of the soundtrack to the movie *Shrek*, and have made it almost an hour into our journey when Madeleine informs us that she has to go to the bathroom. A part of me wants to do a little celebration—for once, we are making an emergency bathroom stop for someone other than me.

I pull off at the next exit, and while Anne and Mike— rookies—scan the terrain for gas stations, I spot the likeliest source for an available public restroom in a nondescript brick building that has a sign outside labeling it a medical office center.

Number one source for public restrooms in an emergency: medical facilities of any sort. They are usually spotlessly clean, and—although I have never been questioned—I presume they would show understanding for anyone needing a bathroom as a result of an IBD emergency. Second best source: large hotels. They have no way to keep track of who belongs in the hotel, and public restrooms are always available somewhere in the lobby. If questioned, you are meeting a friend staying at the hotel. Third best source: fast-food restaurants. The teenage kids behind the counter at McDonald's don't care whether or not you have actually purchased a burger and fries before you use their bathroom.

So I pull into the parking lot, assuring Anne she will find what Madeleine needs inside. Anne doesn't believe me, but she leads Madeleine away by the hand and returns in a few minutes with a small grudging smile on her face.

"I guess I should trust the expert on bathrooms," she says, as she straps Madeleine back into her car seat.

In another forty-five minutes we are driving slowly through traffic in the town of Gloucester, searching for Good Harbor beach. After a stop at a visitor information center, we find it and, arms laden with beach supplies, weave our way through the crush of bodies in the sand and settle into a spot ten yards from the water's edge.

The girls want to go swimming, of course. They love the water, as I do, and will hop into a pool, a lake, or the ocean at every possible chance. So Anne and Mike settle down to spread out our stuff while I follow the girls, who run flapping through the sand, down to the water. I wade into the shallows just behind them.

Oh my God.

I have never felt colder water in my life. I feel like I have stepped into an icy cooler full of beer and soda at someone's backyard barbecue. Within seconds of placing my feet into the water, my toes start to hurt. The girls have walked just a few feet ahead of me, and for a moment I wonder whether their love for the water will overcome their basic human need to keep their bodies warm. I have seen them jump and swim happily in hotel pools that to me seemed frigid.

But I am not imagining this. They turn to me, smiling but surprised, lifting their feet out of the water and squealing. They dash back onto the sand, and then make little forays into the breaking waves, perhaps hoping that the water washing into the shore will bring warmer temperatures.

"Girls," I tell them, "I don't think we're going to be doing much swimming today."

We are all disappointed, perhaps me most thoroughly. They will find other ways to entertain themselves at the beach, and they are probably convinced that the water will warm up eventually. I know better, and I know too how difficult it will be to occupy their attention for an entire day with sand castles.

But we have driven all the way here, and we have to make the best of it, so we settle down a dozen feet from the shoreline and begin building: a moat, surrounded by a great wall; a pyramid in the center covered with rocks, towers at its four base corners. We work diligently for a little while, but their attention begins to wander, and they occasionally make little forays into the water, still expecting to find the water temperature more friendly.

After an hour or so of sand play I decide that I have to brave the water myself, and so I take off my shirt, inform Anne that she is in charge of the girls, and step into the water.

Oh my God.

This time I do my best to shake off the numbing pain in my toes, and move cautiously out into the deeper waters. The ice crawls slowly up my leg: shin, knee, up my thighs and then pauses just below my waist. I am not sure I can stand the agonizing creep of the ice up my genitals, so I have reached the point at which I need either to retreat or to plunge into the surf, submerging the upper half of my body in one fell swoop.

Last summer I would have retreated. I would have seen no good reason to continue to endure the pain in my feet, for the clamp of the icy water around my thighs, for the whole silly experience.

This summer I am a different person. I am hungry now, hungry for experience and sensation in a way that I have never been in my life. I am healthy; I am free of the disease's constraints for the moment, and I want to cram all the life I can into this period of health, because I know it cannot last.

Earlier this past summer, at a swimming pool with some friends in Chicago, I had climbed up thirty feet of winding stairs to a ten-meter diving platform, dizzy and scared, and forced myself to walk off the edge of it and plummet into the diving pool below. As I stood a few feet back from the edge of the platform, I thought my heart would burst out of my chest, or that I would succumb to the weakness in my legs and fall to the platform floor. I could not even look down; I walked off the edge as if I were stepping off a curb and did not see the water until I opened my eyes ten feet deep into it, feet and hands painful and stinging from slapping the water so forcefully.

At the surface I could not help but laugh; it had been terrifying and painful, but I was glad to have done it. I could not remember the last time my nerves and senses had been so intensely alert—the last time I had felt so purely alive.

Standing in the surf, I recollect that moment at the top of the platform, and make my decision. I bend slightly at the knees, and leap into an oncoming wave.

I am confused at first, because I believe someone—someone who must have been waiting for me under the water—has taken a board and slapped me on the chest and face with it. The wind has been knocked out of me, I am gasping for breath, and I can feel the numbing cold, the aftereffects of the slap of that wooden board, on every inch of the surface of my body.

I stand quickly, the water just above my waist, and regain my senses. No one has slapped me; I dove into a sheet of icy water, and it took my breath away. I lower myself into the water to my shoulders, expecting to feel some diminution of the temperature shock the second time around. If there is diminution, I don't feel it.

However hungry I am for new experiences, I have had enough of this one. I turn and walk to the beach, my pace quickening as I near the water's edge. The girls are still at it in the sand, filling buckets with the frigid water and vainly attempting to create a moat, seemingly unfazed by the rapidity with which the sand soaks up each bucketful.

"Grab your buckets," I say, "and let's see what we can find along the beach."

I lead them down the beach, toward the high outcropping of rocks at the far end, a picturesque house perched at their pinnacle.

The shells are few and far between; we run into other families with the same intention we have, and there are simply too many collectors and not enough crustaceans. But we get lucky occasionally. The girls are not as picky as I am; I want them only to collect the best shells, perfectly formed. They are content with scraps and pieces, half-shells and discarded crab legs.

As we approach the end of the beach area, I notice that a small tidal creek runs along the edge of the beach into the sea from a salt marsh back inland. I shepherd the girls toward it. Along the creek I see two boys fishing in the water with nets, and I am curious. I approach them, and kneel down to see what they are seeking and what they have found.

"What're you guys doing?" I ask them.

"Catching crabs," they say. "See?" One of them points me into the bucket they have, which is indeed filled with tiny green crabs, climbing around in a clump of sea vegetation.

I watch them catch the crabs. They sweep their nets into the long strands of green and reddish vegetation that, I now see, fills the edges of the creek. They dump the contents of their nets onto the sand behind them, and invariably they find these little crabs crawling around in the stuff. They grab the crabs in their fat little fingers and deposit them in their buckets.

"Girls! Girls!" I shout to Katie and Madeleine, who are thirty feet away, digging in the shallow surf for something. "Come here, quick!"

They come sprinting over, impressed by the excitement in my voice.

"Look," I say, pointing into the bucket. Just then, one of the boys drops a newly caught load of vegetation onto the sand, and we watch as he sifts through it, searching for crabs. We see an abundance of other creatures there as well: tiny, swimming, millipede-like crustaceans, who crawl around frantically in the leafy material.

Madeleine squats over the vegetation and fingers one of the little creatures intently; I want to warn her that they might bite, but I settle for a more generic warning: "Be careful." I don't want to scare her away from animals, and, besides, they don't look like biters to me.

Katie, in the meantime, can hardly contain her excitement; she is literally hopping up and down as she tugs on my arm.

"Can we get a net, Dad? Did we bring any nets?"

We don't have any nets, so instead we attach ourselves to the boys, becoming their helpers as they continue to forage for marine life in the creek. Katie alternates between tending to the bucket, watching the little crabs, and encouraging the boys in their netting forays. Madeleine is not sure which interests her more, either: the process of catching things in a net, or the animals they find.

I spy Anne walking toward us from the other end of the beach, and I run to within shouting distance.

"Get the stuff!" I yell to her. "Bring it all down here!"

She can see the buckets and nets, and can guess the source of the excitement, so she and Mike dutifully collect our belongings and bring them down by the corner of the beach between the creek and the water line.

In the meantime—and it happens so gradually that it takes me close to an hour to realize it—the tide is going out. The creek has lost five or six feet of width, and at least a foot or two of depth. I step into the edge of it and notice, as well, that it has become warmer, at least at the edges. A cold current still flows through the deepest part of it at the center, but the edges are warm and pleasant.

The girls and I now begin foraging on our own. We grab clumps of the floating vegetation and pull it from the water onto the beach, where we make our own discoveries of tiny crabs and other creatures. Anne has brought us our own buckets, and we fill them with our finds.

One of the clutches of vegetation we pull up brings an incredible treasure: a live starfish. We can't believe our good fortune. I pick it up gently, and find it soft and knobby, yielding at least the surface of its body to the touch. It reacts slowly to our hands, curling its legs around the underside of my hand as I hold it in my palm. I pass it gently to Katie and Madeleine, who stroke it and admire it and then deposit it into our bucket, more excited about the prospect of other new animals than they are about this actual new animal.

The tide has now moved far out to sea. The creek is no more than two or three feet deep in the center, and perhaps a half-dozen feet across in most places. I notice that the water level has sunk below the stony ground at the base of the high rock outcroppings that mark the end of the beach, and tidal pools are forming. I notice, too, that this area of the beach has come alive with people, most of them small children with buckets, supervised by parents who help them find and collect the small animals that are scuttling about in their suddenly exposed environment.

I take the girls' hands and pull them through the creek over to the rocky tidal pools; Mike and Anne join us over there, and we see now that we have happened upon a treasure trove of collectible creatures. With the exception of our starfish friend, we had been pretty limited to small, flat-backed, greenish crabs, and those tiny millipede-like creatures. In these tidal pools we have more than doubled the number of species in our range: we find small, almost transparent, shrimplike creatures, hiding in the sand and darting away swiftly at any disturbance in the water; hermit crabs, from fingernail-sized to as large as an inch or two across the shell; snails and mollusks, clinging fiercely to the wet rocks; and several varieties of small fish, flashing back and forth in the small spaces of the tidal pools, seemingly in search of exits to the sea that the receding tide has closed to them.

Initially I help Katie and Madeleine with their collecting, but eventually I wander away from them and let Anne work with the girls. Mike has strolled off down the creek toward the ocean, and I am left to search through the rocks by myself. Ostensibly I am in search of another starfish; we had shown our earlier one to the two boys, and somehow it found its way into their bucket as they were leaving.

In reality, I am consumed by the same fascination with this eco-system that has infected my daughters. Growing up in the Midwest, I never had such easy exposure to wildlife, though I was fascinated by animals well into my teenage years. My early career dreams, before I understood how academic disciplines like chemistry and physics stood in my way, centered upon fields like veterinary medicine, marine biology, or herpetology (I had a long-standing and inexplicable interest in snakes).

That fascination with the natural world faded and nearly disappeared while I was in college, and throughout most of my twenties. So intent was I upon the world of literature and writing and thinking that I often ignored the external world around me, especially the natural world. Seven years in urban and suburban Chicago, too, throughout graduate school and the first three years of my academic career, limited the possible exposure I might have had to wildlife.

But in recent months I have felt that childhood fascination with the natural world resurge forcefully. The ground for that resurgence had been slowly prepared over the past several years, as my daughters reached the age at which most small children, I think, become fascinated with the other living creatures that surround us in this world. I couldn't help but catch part of their enthusiasm for the natural world.

After my stay in the hospital, in the months that followed and eventually opened up into summer, my interest in nature increased exponentially. I began to take the children on nature walks to the various parks around where we lived; I bought the first field guides I had ever owned, and carted them with me on bike trips through the woods, or on hikes in the local Audubon Society wildlife preserves, or on trips just like this one, to the local beaches. I bought and read nonfiction books on the natural world, and began watching nature specials on television in the evenings with Anne and the girls.

But I have not yet had time to reflect upon what has spurred this interest. Crouched among the tidal pools, some understanding of that begins to press its way to the surface of my mind. I reach into a small tidal pool and pick up a green crab, careful to avoid the small pincers that probably couldn't do me much harm, and set it on a rock a few feet away from the water. The crab momentarily searches for a rock to back under, but then changes tactics and turns hurriedly toward another pool, just a foot or so behind it. The crab's movements seem awkward, jerky—he is clearly more at home in the water—but they impel him along nonetheless, and he finds his watery destination.

Twenty feet away from me Anne leans over to touch and observe something Katie holds in her hand, while Madeleine squats beside them, trolling her finger through a tidal pool. Mike, a nature lover of much longer vintage than myself, has wandered up the creek into the ocean water, following his own interests in this world at the edge of the sea. Around me children are everywhere scrambling over rocks, splashing their feet in small pools, and shouting excitedly to the parents they are towing behind them. At

my feet crabs scuttle about in search of shelter and food, shrimp
and fish dart and flash in the sun, snails and mollusks suck diligently at the moss-covered rocks in the water.

Everywhere, life.

One could stand at the edge of this ocean, in complete soli-
tude, and see only the gentle crashing of the surf against the sand.
But come on a sunny summer day, take just a moment to peer into
these waters, and life appears everywhere—life animal, life plant,
life human; life multicolored, multiformed, multimotile; life that
swims, crawls, hops, scuttles, clings, walks, oozes.

Life that has existed on this planet for hundreds of millions of
years, that has existed in some of these very same forms for at least
that long, and that will continue to exist in these same forms—we
hope—for many more hundreds of millions of years. Life that mul-
tiplies, life with appetites, life that senses, life that seeks to survive
at all costs, against all odds. Life that possesses such infinite variety
and diversity it can exceed our capacity either to understand it or
to appreciate its beauty.

I am no wide-eyed, naive observer of nature. Stay here long
enough, and you will see these creatures devour one another alive;
follow enough of these children around and you will find one of
them pulling the claws off of every crab he can find; cut open these
snails and you will find parasites that have drilled into their shells
and curled deep within their intestines, siphoning off their food.

But even these aspects of life are part of the cycle, and do not
slow or deter nature's creatures from their basic drives to produce
and reproduce new life. My still superficial readings in the literature of the natural world have conveyed one lesson to me more
clearly than anything else: Living things seek, first and foremost,
survival and reproduction. The goal of life is to produce more
life—however scarred, however transformed, however sickened by

that life's encounters with this world, with its own genetic defects, and with its own mortality. Life pulses on.

In my understanding of that fundamental fact, in the basic evidence of it that I have come to see in the natural world around me, in my reflections on it—on a warm August day, crouched in the tidal pools of Gloucester, Massachusetts, with my wife and children and my friend—I have begun to take comfort. I have begun to see my own life's place within these larger cycles, and to see connections between my struggle for life and health and the struggles for life and health of so many of earth's creatures around me.

Between the sea and the sky, my feet moistened in the water and my back baked by the sun, I feel the force of life pulsing within me, too. I feel strong and resilient, the survivor of a year in which my body has ravaged itself for no reason that anyone can fully understand. I have shat and bled and wept my way through a terrible year, but I have scratched and clawed my way to this moment of health and happiness, and I have my wife and my children and my friends and my God intact along with me.

Whatever happens to me in two weeks, in two months, in two years, I have this moment to hang onto, this moment of both joy and wisdom. Without having experienced what I have undergone this year, I am certain I would let this moment slip away— unnoticed, unmarked, and unremembered. Instead, it is etching its way into my body and my brain, and it is a moment to which I know I shall return, again and again, in the years to come.

THE SUN HAS BEGUN its descent toward the horizon, and we want to spend an hour or two wandering through the tents and makeshift shops of the Gloucester Waterfront Festival, a mile or so from the beach. Reluctantly, the girls spill their buckets into the tidal pools, and we watch as the small animals find their way back to their homes in the water and the waves.

Slowly we return to our blankets and cooler, and slowly we gather everything up and trek over the sand back to our car. We cleanse ourselves briefly in the beach's outdoor showers, and pack our belongings into the minivan.

At the Waterfront Festival we wander in and out of the tents that are selling an incredible variety of handmade gifts and household items, occasionally purchasing the things that catch our eyes: Mike buys some pieces of driftwood painted with New England lighthouses, and Anne and I pick out some dried starfishes for the girls. They will end up atop the bookshelves in our family room, where they sit to this day. Further along, we let the girls fill small bags with the colorful shells an older woman is selling; useful material, I am certain, for a future project.

Tired of walking, we return to the car and drive along the harbor until we spot a restaurant that looks promising: Mr. T's Lobster House. Inside we settle down and I order a beer. It tastes good, absolutely perfect after a day in the sun and an hour or two of slow strolling. I can feel a good sort of tiredness creeping up on me, the sort that will enable me to sleep well tonight.

The menu contains all sorts of things I would like to order— especially a steak dish that I saw someone eating as we made our way through the restaurant to our table. But I settle, instead, for tuna shish kebab. I try to order fish, now, as much as possible when we are eating out. I stopped taking the fish oil tablets that I had read about as helpful for Crohn's disease in a nutrition book earlier that year; I couldn't stand the fact that I would be belching salmon for an hour or two after I took them, twice a day. So I try to get as much fish oil as I can naturally.

Unfortunately, I have never really liked fish all that much. But this dinner is delicious, and afterward I am happy and proud that I ordered and ate what I should have.

We make the long ride back to Worcester mostly in silence; Mike sits beside me in the passenger seat, and we talk occasionally about the upcoming school year. The girls are sleeping in their car seats, and Anne, in the far backseat, is nodding in and out herself.

Back at home, after depositing Mike at his apartment, we carry the girls into their beds and change them into their pajamas, still asleep. We pick up the toys they had managed to pull out before we had left that morning, and I am preparing to sit down and read or watch television in the family room.

"You know," Anne says to me, "I'm two weeks late at this point."

It has been nearly five months since my release from the hospital, and we have not yet had any luck with conceiving another child. Anne was initially concerned that perhaps my illness, or the medications I have been taking, have hurt her chances of becoming pregnant.

In the late spring we saw a fertility specialist. We explained my situation, and they arranged the appropriate tests for me. When we returned a week or two later, the news was good; I was still perfectly capable of impregnating Anne. That left more tests for Anne, which showed an irregularity in the way in which eggs were being produced in her cycle. She began taking a drug to regulate her cycle, and to receive an injection just prior to her most fertile time of the month.

But our summer travels had twice, in the last two months, prevented her from getting this injection at the right time, so we had essentially put our hopes on hold until we could return from our vacations and settle into our normal life in September.

"Do you have any pregnancy tests?"

"I have a two-pack upstairs."

I can tell she is reluctant, she doesn't want to find out for certain; if she doesn't take the test, she might still be pregnant. If she takes it and finds it negative, it means another month of waiting.

"Well, go take one!"

She heads upstairs, and I hear her opening the package and then closing the bathroom door. A minute later she comes downstairs.

"Well?"

"You have to wait two minutes," she says. "I can't look. You go up there and check."

So I go up there, but I don't go into the bathroom yet. She said it would take two minutes, so I go and sit on the bed. I have a momentary flash of all that a third child will bring us, good and bad: more diapers, more crying, more late nights and too-early mornings; more little tiny fingers, more smiles and laughter, more opportunities to help a small human being learn to negotiate the world.

Anne calls up the stairs to me.

"Well?"

"It hasn't been two minutes yet."

She walks back into the kitchen. I sit for another minute, and then take the short walk to the bathroom. Sitting on the counter I see the white plastic wand that holds the answer to our question.

I pick it up, and see it there, in the small window: a pink cross. Pregnant.

"Anne," I call downstairs. "Come up here and see for yourself."

She hurries upstairs and I show her. We embrace, and we both shed a few tears.

"Finally," I say.

"Finally," she says.

AND THAT MUST BE HOW this story ends, with the two of us once again locked in an embrace, once again with tears in our eyes, but in a situation so far removed from that embrace in the basement twelve months ago that I can hardly believe such extremes are possible in a single human life.

Those two embraces mark the opening and closing of a year that I have vowed never to forget. That first embrace carried me through seven months of illness and depression; this second embrace represents everything that has become valuable to me in the five months that have brought me to this instant in Anne's arms.

No one on this earth can predict how long this period of health and happiness will last for me, for us, but I banish that thought from my mind as soon as it enters.

Suspend this moment, frozen in time, and leave us here, now, locked in one another's arms, new life forming between us, and this moment—for just a moment—the only thing that matters in the world.

EPILOGUE

The Cardinal Rules for Crohn's Disease

The wisdom that I have gained over the course of the year described in this book is impossible for me to distill into an easy list of lessons. The lessons—about life with illness, about life with a physical self, about life as a human being—are too firmly embedded in the experiences I describe to rip them out of context and place them in a form that I think will reduce them to platitudes.

I do believe, though, that I learned some very specific lessons about the handling of chronic illness in general, and Crohn's disease in particular, and that those lessons might be usefully reiterated here for those readers who are struggling with their own chronic illnesses, or those of loved ones. I offer these especially to the newly diagnosed, with the hope that they can learn these lessons more easily and quickly than the year of illness it took me to absorb them into my body and my brain.

1. **Accept the presence of the disease in your life.** Do not expect God, or modern medicine, or any other substitute

for these entities, to cure you. Hope for a cure, pray for a cure, raise funds for a cure, campaign for public awareness for a cure—*but do not put your life on hold waiting for one.* Learn what accommodations you must make to the disease in your life; make those accommodations; get on with your life.

2. **Act quickly.** Learn the patterns of your disease, and become familiar with the signals that indicate an oncoming flare. When you can see those symptoms appearing, call your doctor *immediately*. Intervene as early as possible in order to prevent flares from spiraling out of control.

3. **Become your own patient advocate.** Not only can doctors not cure this disease; they cannot even yet tell us what causes it. Visit three different doctors and you might receive three different recommendations for treatment. Do not let doctors—or nurses, or dietitians, or your friends or families—make your medical decisions for you. Buy every book you can find, read as much scientific jargon as you can tolerate, and educate yourself about the human body and this disease. *Play an active role in your medical care.*

4. **Learn when to live and when to rest.** We are both blessed and cursed with a disease that comes and goes, and can spin us from remission into the hospital and back into remission again in the course of a few months. When you are healthy, *live intensely*. Gather sensation and experience as greedily as you can. When you are sick, rest and attend to your body. Although you may lose sight of this when you are in the middle of months or years of illness, a time will come again when you are healthy.

5. **Tell your story.** Tell it for yourself, first. We make sense of our lives through the stories we tell about ourselves. Telling

the story of your disease—on paper, on the Internet, to a friend—will help you see the disease's place in your life more clearly. Tell it for your friends and families, second. They need—and in most cases want—to understand what you are going through. Tell it, finally, for the rest of the world. Research funding and increasingly sophisticated medical care will increase with greater public awareness of the disease.

Resources for Crohn's Disease and Ulcerative Colitis

❧

M y methods of gathering information about Crohn's disease were quirky and unsystematic, as most people's probably will be; usually when you most need information about the disease, you are in no position to expend the energy you would need to find it. Over the years, as I had more time to devote to my research, I have managed to put together a more comprehensive picture of those resources.

Most people, in their initial search for information, will turn to the World Wide Web. Be careful. The first sites that come up in some search engines are from people or organizations that are trying to sell you something. Do not be misled by any site promising you a complete cure for your disease—there is *no* cure for this disease at this time. Do not change your medications, or your diet, or your life without at least hearing the opinion of your doctor about whatever you have read.

But the Web can obviously be an excellent source of information as well, and it can provide you with opportunities to connect with others with Crohn's disease. Those connections—whether they take place in person, through support groups; online, through chat rooms; or on paper, through books—can be essential to maintaining your sanity and helping you see your own disease in perspective.

I offer here the top three resources that I turn to most frequently when I am in need of information, of help, and of support. These three resources are well-established and available at the time of publication, and I expect they will remain so as you are reading this book.

Crohn's and Colitis Foundation of America (CCFA)
386 Park Avenue South, 17th Floor
New York, NY 10016
Phone: 800-932-2423
Fax: 212-779-4098
Web: www.ccfa.org

Stop here first. The CCFA can provide you with information, with links to a plenitude of other resources, and with assistance in finding a physician. The CCFA funds research on the disease, and advocates for legislation to improve the quality of life for IBD sufferers. Join the organization to receive their newsletters, and donate to it at least a part of your budget earmarked for charity. Ten percent of the author's proceeds from this book will be donated to the CCFA.

Sklar, Jill, *The First Year: Crohn's Disease and Ulcerative Colitis.* New York: Marlowe, 2002.

I have found this book, authored by a medical writer with Crohn's disease, to provide the most easily accessible and up-to-date information on everything related to the disease: causes, symptoms, medications and their side effects, diet and nutrition, psychological issues. The book's table of contents provides easy access to information in just about every imaginable area related to inflammatory bowel disease.

IBD Sucks Web Forum: www.ibdsucks.org

Operated by Bill Robertson, this irreverently named Web site offers the opportunity to chat with fellow sufferers around the globe about everything related to IBD—and I mean everything. Those terrible and embarrassing parts of the disease that you thought you could never share with anyone? You'll find folks talking about that stuff here. In general, I have found the users of this site friendly and knowledgeable about the disease; posters often provide abstracts of current articles in medical journals, or links to other useful resources. A massive index directs you to conversation threads in literally dozens of specific areas. I go to this site when I'm feeling sorry for myself, and I usually feel better afterward.

. . . and, of course . . .

Learning Sickness Web Site: www.learningsickness.com

Read the comments of others who have read this book, post your own comments, and keep up with the author's progress and thoughts on chronic illness. The Web site also offers a fuller—and continually updated—list of links and Web resources.